The Beginner's guide to Essential Oil Making

All the secrets for successful enfleurage and distillation,
40 detailed plant sheets

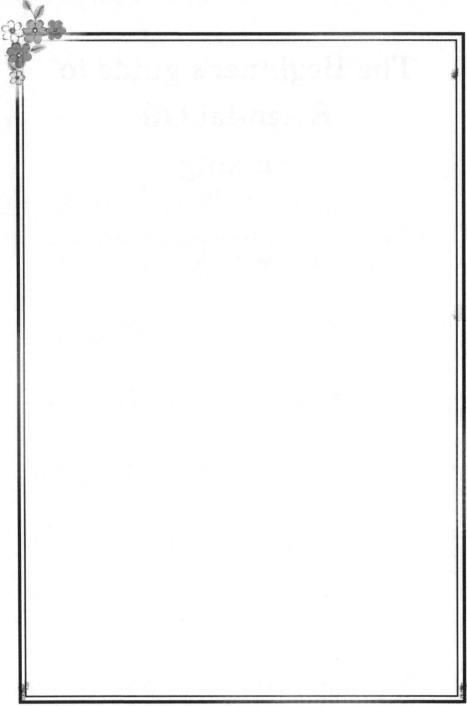

Table of contents:

Preamble:

An essential oil is an odorant product, with a complex chemical composition, obtained from a raw plant material.

The virtues of essential oils no longer need to be demonstrated. Since ancient times, they have been used as remedies (ingested, inhaled or applied topically during massages), cosmetics, sanitizers, or even perfumes...

In this book, after having gone through the fascinating history of oil distillation, we will pick the plants from which they are extracted. We will learn how to prepare them properly, while discovering their properties and particularities. Then we will immerse ourselves in the age-old art of distillation and the almost magical use of a still. Finally, we will learn how to extract the essence of these plants when distillation is impossible (enfleurage, cold-pressing...).

I - A brief history of distillation

1. Antiquity: Alchemy in its infancy

It is difficult to date the appearance of the first still precisely. The earliest evidence dates to the Babylonian era when the first distillations would have been carried out in skilful pottery systems. The mixture is placed in the heart of an earthenware vessel over a fire. A clay lid on top collects the vapours that condense on its surface into water droplets: these trickle down its length before being collected by an ingenious double-edged groove system. Although they do not specifically describe the distillation process, the alchemical tablets in the British Museum in London give us recipes in cuneiform writing that give us a good idea of their know-how. A recipe for counterfeiting a precious stone has come down to us:

"Bring the alum to the boil and [...] in the vinegar. Place the stone in the lapis-lazulis coloured liquid. You will obtain a 'dušû' coloured stone."

Aware of its importance, the Babylonian scholarly elite jealously guarded its alchemical knowledge. Fortunately for us, Persian merchants brought this alchemical know-how to the Egypt of the Pharaohs. In the darkness of their temples, the Pharaonic priests tried their hand at making substitutes for gold, silver and precious pigments. From there, the knowledge was passed on to the Greeks in the early centuries before Christ, during the Hellenistic period. They interpreted the works of the Pharaohs according to their own representation of nature and the elements. Thus, Aristotle asserted as early as the IVe century BC that Greek sailors could desalinate sea water by a method of condensation of vapours (distillation).

Let's stay on the warm and green shores of the Nile. The year is 300 AD. The Roman Empire dominates the Mediterranean. A scientist, **Zosimus of Panopolis**, is about to revolutionise chemistry. Zosimus learns (according to some authors) alchemy in Alexandria, Egypt, and travels throughout the country to perfect his knowledge and design the first contemporary alembic. Thanks to a carefully copied manuscript from the 17th century, a trace of the object remains. Was he inspired by the Greeks, Indians or Egyptians for his still? We do not know, but his name and his work marked a turning point in the history of distillation.

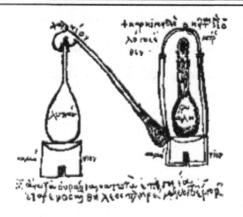

Zosime distillation apparatus,
Parisinus graecus 2325 fol. 81v

Radically different from vase systems with capitals, the Zosimus still has four distinct parts:

- **the cucurbit** (*lopas*) placed over the fire and containing the mixture to be distilled.

- **the capital** (*phialè*) whose name will give the flask, in charge of collecting and condensing the vapours.

- **the pipe** (*solen*) for collecting the distillate.

- **a container** (*bicos*).

This device allows for the very first time to distil the product without the vapours falling back into the water, thanks to the *solen* which collects them and directs them towards the *bicos*. It is worth

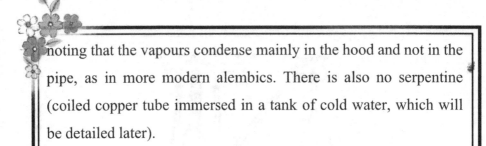

noting that the vapours condense mainly in the hood and not in the pipe, as in more modern alembics. There is also no serpentine (coiled copper tube immersed in a tank of cold water, which will be detailed later).

2.   Arab civilisation and distillation of oils

Alchemy: from *Al-Chimie*, Arabic transposition of Greek χημεία (Chēmea, cheo, to melt), from Accadian *kamû* (to cook, to burn): one who seeks to *transmute materials,* or from Egyptian *Kem-Et* (black soil).

In the 7th century AD, Arab horsemen left their cradle in Saudi Arabia to take over an empire stretching from Andalusia to the borders of Persia. This was the golden age of Islamic civilisation and of Arab scholars. The Caliph Al-Mamoun founded the House of Wisdom, a place dedicated to the sciences where works were brought from Constantinople. Within this ebullition of sciences, alchemy was not left out.

It is likely that it was during the annexation of Persia in the 7th century that the alchemical know-how of ancient civilisations was passed on to them. Not content with reproducing the experiments of their predecessors, they translated the apocryphal ancient texts and attempted to mathematise the composition of matter and chemical reactions. Great names followed one another, led by **Jabbir Ibn Hayyan** (Geber). Born in Iraq and son of a pharmacist, Geber developed a passion for alchemy at an early age. He perfected Zosimus' alembic and discovered hydrochloric and nitric acids. He was the first to classify the substances into several categories: those that vaporise in a flame, those that are crushed (stones), and metals. Finally, he wrote "*Kitab al-Kîmia*" (the book of chemistry), translated by Robert of Castre for the major European universities. It is from these translations that we inherit the terms:

- Alembic: *Al-Anbiq*, which describes the shape of their stills.
- Elixir: *Al-Iksir*, which means "the fraction".

Moreover, still in the field of etymology, alcoholic beverages are called "*Al-Araq*" (sweat), which is remarkable when we know that the Latin root of the word "distillation" (*distillatio*) translates as "to flow from drop to drop". The term alcohol has a more convoluted etymology since the term "*Al-Khôl*", meaning the fine thing, was in fact antimony sulphide used for eye make-up (the famous Khôl). It was not until centuries later that brandy was called "alcohol". [1]

---

[1] It was often prestigious for medieval authors to insert 'Al-' as a prefix to a word or character.

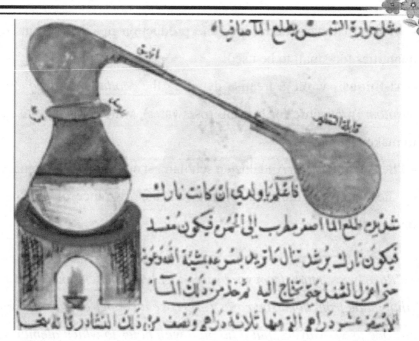

"Then you bring the mixture to a very low heat. If [the product that comes out] is red in colour, then it is lost and you will have to start again. If it is yellow, then you have succeeded.

Kitab al Kimiya, 8th century, British Library, Jabbir Ibn Hayan

A single book would be too short to detail all the developments of these scholars around the still. We will simply note that, based on Geber's work, major advances were made, especially in the distillation of plants and the production of essential oils:

- **Al-Kindi** worked on hydraulic distillation (which we will study in the following chapters).

- **Al-Razi** (Rhazes) developed the production of ethanol, but in quantities too small to be used.

- **Al-Buqasis** wrote a treatise detailing the *Modus facien aquam rosatam* (procedure for making rose water), which was later used to make alcohol.

- **The Cordouan,** an Andalusian scholar, set out to study the impact of the quality of the plant on the delicate fragrance of the oils obtained...

"Rose water made from wild roses [...] has a better smell than that made from domestic roses [...]. Take a copper cauldron like the one used by dyers, put a lid on it with holes to which alembics can be fitted, fill the cauldron with water and light a fire underneath with vine shoots and distil. When the distillation is halfway through, you must cover the furnace until the distillation is finished. And to whoever wants to put coals instead of wood, the water will be more fragrant." - Al-Buqasi

3.   The Middle Ages: discovery of spirit

A founding date of alchemy in Europe is 1148, when Robert de Castres translated Geber's works. Western universities quickly took up the process and added their stone to the edifice.

Among the biggest names:

- **The pseudo-Geber,** Paul of Taranto, developed the regal water, *aqua regia*, capable of melting gold, by mixing two volumes of hydrochloric acid in one volume of nitric acid.
- **Albert the Great**, a man of the cloth, also embarked on the alchemical adventure. He demonstrated the interesting properties of Cinable (red stone or *lapis rubens*), composed of sulphur and mercury. He described the preparation of nitric acid, "philosophical water in its first degree of perfection", which made it possible to separate silver from gold. His discoveries made him one of the greatest medieval alchemists.
- **Thomas Aquinas**, a disciple of Albert the Great, reports on the techniques for making counterfeit gems and colouring crystals.

It was also during this period that **water of life** was developed. Although Arab scholars had already discovered its existence earlier, they had not been able to extract enough of it. Thus, in an innovative text, Taddeo Alderotti proposed a new method of distillation in which **the still was connected to a coil** around which cold water circulated, allowing for accelerated cooling. This *serpentis* distillation technique made it possible to distil *aqua ardens* (the water that provides flames), to purify it into *aqua vitae*, "eau de vie" in French (spirit), and then to purify it further into *aqua perfecta* and *aqua perfectissima* (probably 90° alcohol). This was the discovery of alcohol, made according to the same processes as those described by the Arabs for distilling rose water! It is by the way reported:

"Sic fit aqua rosacea, et exibit per sublimationes aqua ardens"
As rose water is made, so sublimate ardent water.

This discovery upset contemporary chemical representations. According to the Aristotelian tradition, there are only "four elements that Friendship gathers and Hate separates". Fire, air, water, earth. Four distinct elements that cannot coexist: and yet *aqua ardens* is water that catches fire! When a sheet is immersed in it, it can catch fire without being consumed. To solve this dilemma, John of Rupescissa, a Franciscan monk, proposed to create the *quinta essencia*, the fifth essence, the purest product of distillation.

It was soon realised that *aqua ardens* prevents or delays the putrefaction of bodies. It was then attributed the greatest virtues. It purges the liver and stomach, cures nervous disorders, and is used in all pharmacopoeias. As the quantities produced were relatively small, its domestic use only became more widespread later, around the 15th century, when it was first used in recipes for making spiced wines such as *hypocras* or pastries with alcohol. Distillation was no longer reserved for the rich and powerful lords, or for a few mad scientists in their tower. It also benefited the people.

4.   From renaissance to chemistry

"Many people have inquired whether alchemy is really capable of making gold; but that does not matter. It is the foundation and the pillar of all medicine. Without it, no one has the right to call himself a doctor."

Paracelsus, 16th century

Far from being a rediscovery of science after a long phase of ignorance and obscurantism, the renaissance was a continuation of the discoveries of previous centuries. It marked the beginning of a change in the approach to science. Caught between rationalism and occult traditions, many currents of thought clashed. The same authors mixed scientific experimentation with magical thinking.

On a more scientific level, we will remember above all the name of **Paracelsus**, who gave alchemy an impetus and a medical objective. He produced remedies from plants such as antimony. Georges Aricola dealt with metals and Bécher invented the beaker, which is still used today in chemistry.

It was finally Francis Bacon, Boyle and Descartes who stripped alchemy of all its mystical beliefs in the following centuries, opening the way to Chemistry...

II - Essential Oils

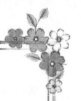

1. Definition

"Essential Oil: An odorous product, of complex composition, obtained from a botanically defined plant raw material."

European Pharmacopoeia

Essential oils are derived from chemical components naturally present in plants and extracted in various ways (most often by distillation). All parts of plants are likely to contain oils: from flowers to roots, tree gums, rhizomes, bulbs... Most often, oils are present in very small quantities in plants, except in the case of aromatic plants, where the contents are higher (less than 10% of species). There are four secretory organs:

- **Isolated secretory cells**: mainly on the plant surface.
- **Secretory hairs**: like a hair (made of one cell) with a secretory cell on top.
- **Secretory pockets**: pockets made of secretory cells, where the essence accumulates, very present in the leaves of the Eucalyptus.
- **Secretory ducts**: duct paved with secretory cells.

Why do plants produce oils? We don't really know yet, but there are many clues. They could be a way for the plant to protect itself against pathogens (bacteria, microbes, fungi). In some cases, they can attract insect pollinators. They mediate with the plants' immediate environment (especially with neighbouring plants) and can act as a messenger within the plant.

2. Chemical properties

Some key chemical properties are necessary to understand for the rest of this book.

Essential Oils (EO) are most often **liquid** (with a few exceptions, for example Myrrh EO which is viscous). Of very varied appearance, the name "oil" first recalls their consistency. Be careful, because of the presence of polymerising compounds, if they are left exposed to light and to fresh air, they can denature and become viscous or even solid. You can easily make the experiment: leave a few drops of lavender essential oil in the open air, a few days later it will have a resin-like consistency.

They are **volatile**. They can be carried away by steam (and therefore evaporate easily). This is what distinguishes them from fatty oils, such as olive oil. Pure, EO volatilize when heated and do not leave a stain. It is this property that we will use to separate the oils from the rest of the plant by heat during distillation: we will evaporate the oils contained in the plant material before recovering them by cooling them!

They are generally **lipophilic**: they do not mix with water. This property is interesting because during distillation, a large quantity of floral water (**hydrosol**) is also collected. As the oil is not miscible with the water, we can easily separate it. Here again, beware of exceptions: some molecular compounds extracted from rosemary oil (verbenone) or lavender oil (lavandulol) dissolve in water and will be present in the hydrosol.

Their **colour** is mostly pale yellow. However, some compounds can colour them, such as chamazulene (extracted from Chamomile) which has a blue tint.

Their **density** is in most cases lower than that of water, leading them to float in solutions. Nevertheless, it can happen that their density is very close to or even higher than that of water (cloves, onions, garlic), in which case the extracted oil will sink to the bottom of the containers and an adapted extraction method will have to be used. We will discuss this in more details later.

3. Molecular families

Essential oils contain various molecules, sometimes redundant between plants, which define a signature for each plant.

These molecules can be classified into different families, with specific properties. We can give a non-exhaustive overview:

o **Terpenes:** the main component of many oils, they come in various sub-families:

- Monoterpenes: These molecules have antibacterial, expectorant and inflammatory system stimulating virtues. They are the ones that confer the atmospheric cleansing properties (especially for pine oil, whose resin is rich in them). Among them are mainly limonene, α and β-pinene.
  - ❖ Caution: some Monoterpenes are dermo-caustic (skin irritants) and should be diluted. They can also be toxic for the kidneys (juniper oil).
- Sesqui-terpenic carbides: In plants, they play a role in the defence against pathogens. For example, we find

Chamazulene (EO of Chamomile or Yarrow, of blue colour) which has anti-histaminic, anti-inflammatory and anti-oxidant properties. Farnesol (lemon) is a pesticide and repellent. It is also used as a flavouring agent.

❖ Caution: some are irritating, so dilute them as well.

o **Alcohols and Phenols:** frequently found in oils, they play a stimulating, antibacterial and antifungal role.

• Phenols are powerful anti-infectious agents (Amoxicillin in Augmentin™ contains a phenol nucleus, for example). They are found in essential oils, for example carvacrol (Oregano, Thyme), eugenol (Clove, chilli, cinnamon), or Thymol (Thyme). They also stimulate the brain, and sometimes have hypertensive and excitatory effects.

❖ Caution: they are even more irritating than terpenes and are hepatotoxic (toxic to the liver) in high doses. They can also have effects on blood coagulation.

• Monoterpenols are also good anti-infectious agents. The most frequently encountered is linalool, present in Lavender oil (skin tonic and sedative). Menthol (Mint, vasoconstrictor -contracts the vessels- and hepato-stimulant -stimulates the liver-) is also one of them.

- Sesquiterpenols and Diterpenols are molecules with activities on the endocrine system, with structures close to steroid hormones (oestrogen).

o **Aldehydes:** have mainly a sedative, antihypertensive and calming effect. It is most often these molecules that give certain oils their lemony smell. The best known is Citronelal (Lemongrass, Lemon Verbena, Lemon Balm), a powerful insect repellent.

- Caution: these molecules also have skin irritating effects.

o **Acids:** of various types and classes, the acidic compounds in oils have mainly anti-inflammatory effects. The best example is Salicylic Acid (Aspirin), which has anti-inflammatory and anti-pyretic (fever reducing) properties.

o **Esters:** have mainly spasmolytic properties (reduction of spasms) by action on the nervous system. They are also anti-inflammatory.

o **Ethers:** these molecules have antispasmodic and analgesic effects. Among them: Estragole (Tarragon) and Anethole (Green Anise).

❖ Caution: these molecules are skin irritants and can be responsible for confusion, neurological and respiratory disorders. Particular care must be taken with their storage to avoid an increase in toxicity.

o **Ketones:** these molecules have interesting properties for healing and coagulation. Some of them can allow the resorption of haematomas (Arnica). They have mucolytic activities (Verbenone, Rosemary), and promote biliary secretion (Menthone, Carvone).

❖ Caution: they can also be toxic for the nervous system and extremely harmful for the foetus (therefore, they are not recommended for pregnant women).

o **Terpene oxides:** the main one is 1,8-cineole, found for example in Eucalyptus, with a mucolytic and expectorant effect.

❖ Caution: they can be dermo-caustic.

o **Lactones:** rare in oils (<5%), they can be neurotoxic.

o **Coumarins:** these molecules mainly have effects on coagulation. Although very low in concentration in oils, they are sufficient to interact with treatments (e.g. Coumadin) and the greatest precaution should be observed.

o **Phthalides:** these molecules have a beneficial effect on the liver. They also have aphrodisiac effects.

o **Nitrogenous and sulphurous compounds:** extremely rare in oils in general, they are found in large quantities in garlic or onion essential oil. They have a powerful antibacterial effect.

❖ Caution: they are irritating to the skin.

4. Chemical variability factors of oils

It is important to understand that the same plant species can produce oils of different molecular composition (**different chemotypes**) depending on its location, the type of soil it grows on, its exposure, etc. Thus, even if the molecular profiles will most often be similar, the proportions may change between plants.

Climate: Plants grown in a warm country have the strongest aroma and the highest yield. In temperate climates, the yield is lower, but the aroma will be finer...

Exposure: Exposure can modify the chemotype within the same plant or plants of the same species. For example, for the same Laurel, leaves exposed to the South are more interesting to distil (better yield) than leaves exposed to the North. Similarly, the more Spearmint is exposed to ultraviolet radiation (based on geographical and topographical differences), the more linalool it will contain.

Exposure to rain also alters the oils for the most fragile plants. In the case of Jasmine, the flowers washed by the rain have an altered perfume. They must be cut off to develop the neighbouring buds.

Part of the plant used: Two parts of the same plant can produce oils with different molecular properties. For example, in the case of the orange tree, the leaves, the flowers and the fruits contain different oils. Some parts also contain more oil than others. Again, in the case of the orange tree, it will be very easy to extract the oil from the pericarp of the fruit, whereas the flowers, which have a much subtler fragrance, will require more advanced techniques (enfleurage, which we will discuss in more details later).

Harvest time: Depending on the time of year, plants change their oil content and composition. There is no general rule. Here are some examples to illustrate:

- Menthone is more present in **Peppermint** during the flowering period.

- It is best to extract the essential oil of **Coriander** from the fruit when it is ripe.

- **Lavender** should be harvested when two-thirds of the flowers are open (more esters are present, allowing soap to be made).

- **Sage** should be harvested in winter.

- **Thyme** has its maximum yield in the flowering period.

Time of harvest: As with the time of year, the time of harvest affects oil composition and yield. For example, roses have a better yield if their petals are harvested just after the dew, between 6 and 9 am. Conversely, Carnations should be harvested two or three hours after sunshine. Unfortunately, there are often no precise rules here either. We will give you instructions when they are available, otherwise you will have to try...

The pre-fanning and drying stages: Often useful for increasing yield, these stages also modify the molecular content of the oils (sometimes as desired). For example, drying thyme reduces its oil yield with a loss of thymol. It seems that the best compromise here is to dry **below 40°C (25 to 35°C).**

Thus, if one wanted to be as rigorous as possible, when buying oil, one should have access to the family of the plant, to the part of the plant that has been distilled, but also to its environment. In practice, given the diversity of producers involved in the production of a single bottle of commercial oil, this is not possible. This diversity of confounding factors makes it difficult to standardise production and production methods. It could be said that in general, one should pick:

- Fully opened but not withered flowers
- Leaves and stems when the flowers are about to open
- Ripe fruit

- Roots at the end of Spring

... But there is no exact recipe, **you must try.**

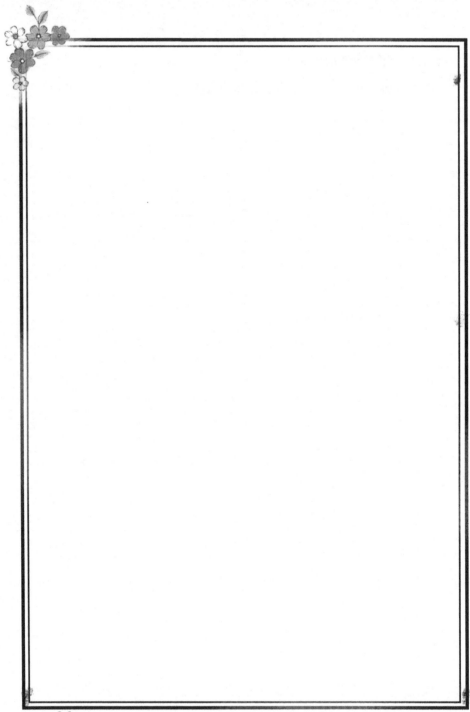

III - Extracting oil from a plant

1. Introduction

There are several ways to extract oil from a plant, the main one being <u>distillation</u>. Distillation consists of **separating different elements by heat**. The various elements are first vaporised into a gas which is then recovered, isolated and condensed to recover a liquid oil. There are many distillation techniques: fractional, under reduced pressure, dry... but we will only focus here on the historical method: **steam distillation**.

In some cases, distillation is not the appropriate method. For the most fragile plants, with heat-sensitive molecules, **enfleurage** should be used to preserve their scent.

Other plants (such as oranges) can release their oil by simple **pressing** or cold extraction, without the need for the whole distillation process (note that the oil produced has different properties).

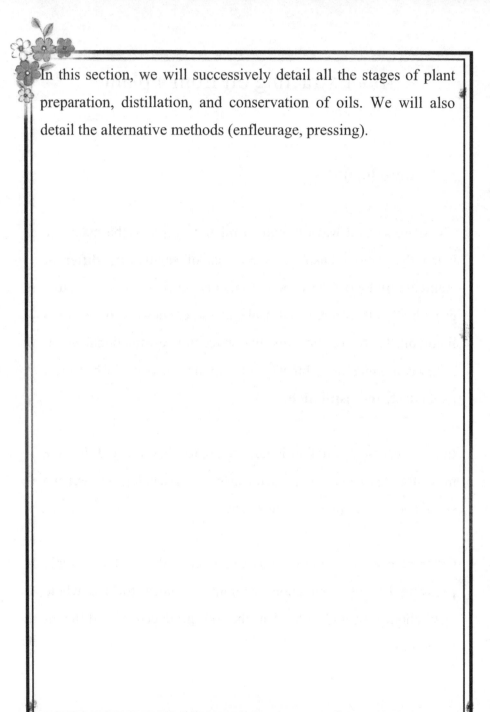

In this section, we will successively detail all the stages of plant preparation, distillation, and conservation of oils. We will also detail the alternative methods (enfleurage, pressing).

2. Preparation: Dry the plants

It is usually best to dry and then finely chop the plant material before distillation. If you have large stems, we advise you to **dry** them upside **down**. The ideal drying temperature is **between 25 and 35°C**. Be sure to place a drip tray under the drying stems in case parts of the plant come off.

Once the leaves are dry, chop them finely. This will maximise the yield and reduce the distillation time.

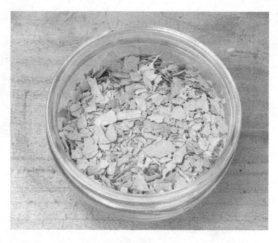

Dried and chopped Eucalyptus leaves

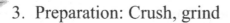

3. Preparation: Crush, grind

A certain number of plants will have to be crushed or ground before being distilled, to increase the yield. This is the case for seeds (cloves) and bark (for example: Cinnamon).

The solution is easy. Instead of dulling the blades of your favourite blender, invest in ... a mallet! Place the plants in a small plastic bag and crush them before distilling.

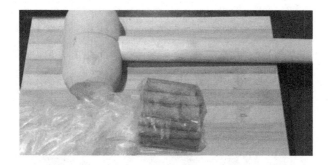

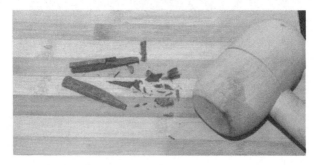

Crushed Cinnamon

4. Preparation: Softwoods

The distillation of softwoods can be tedious. It is essential to carry out a pre-fanning of several days in the open air. Then, the thorns must be chopped open: as the cellular layer on the surface of the leaves is thick, the yield will be negligible without this step. The rest of the distillation process is the same as for the rest of the plants.

First... find a nice pine tree! Let the leaves dry for two to three days upside down.

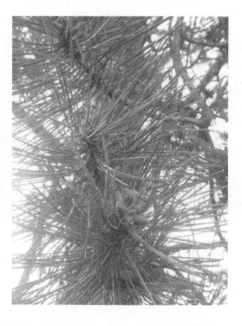

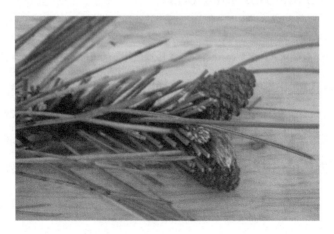

Then remove the twigs from the stem and cut them finely with small secateurs. Chop the result before distilling.

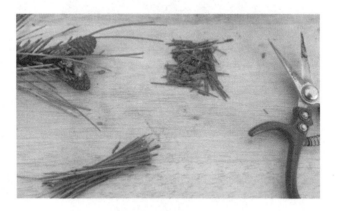

5. Preparation: Citrus fruits

The essential oil of citrus fruits is most often collected by cold pressing. However, it is possible to distil them. To do this, nothing could be easier! Gently peel your orange (lemon, lime, bergamot...), using a peeler.

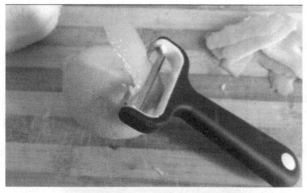

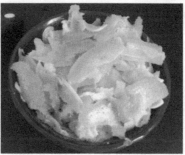

This will give you the zest, which you will then have to chop up. Steam distil the chopped peel, the yield is often very good!

6. Distillation: The different types of stills

The process of steam distillation is always the same: the plant is heated to a sufficient temperature to volatilise its oils, which are then condensed and recovered. This framework can be broken down into different devices, which we will present. Afterwards, we will illustrate a distillation with the traditional still.

- <u>Traditional still</u>

Description and implementation: The round **pot** (cucurbit) is designed to hold vegetal material and water. It is placed above a heat source, ideally gas, whose temperature will be raised gradually. As the mixture rises in temperature, the volatilized vapours and oils condense first in the tulip-shaped **hood** and then in the **swan neck**, before being cooled by the **coil** (see illustration below). The oils and floral water are collected in a glass vial.

Cooling: Cool water (or ice) circulates around the coil. The water should enter from the bottom of the container containing the coil and be discharged from the top. Most often tap water is used with the help of various adapters to connect pipes to the still. To avoid waste, a small water pump (such as an automatic sprinkler) can be used. If the water is in a closed circuit, make sure that the volume of water is sufficient to maintain thermal inertia: if the external water tank is too low, the water will heat up quickly on contact with the coil and the oils will not be cooled properly.

The vapours should be cooled as quickly as possible. If the temperature of the cooling liquid is too high, up to 50% of the fragrance can be lost and the rest will be spoiled!

Avoiding losses: The various joints and gaps between the pieces should be sealed. For this purpose, a Teflon tape or a classic bread dough reconstituted from water and flour can be used (a few spoonfuls of flour and a little water mixed into a dough, without yeast of course!) Finally, a thermometer is an essential accessory for controlling the distillation temperature.

Distillation time: Care should be taken to stop distillation before all the water has evaporated, as this could burn the plant material. From our experience with this still, the best distillations are done with a maximum yield during the first half hour.

Proportions: For flowers, an equivalent mass of water and flowers is sufficient, for leaves we obtained better results with one and a half mass of water per mass of leaves (1.5/1) and a longer distillation time. The best results were obtained when the alembic was 3/4 full. The leaves needs to be cut into small pieces and the whole plant material must be packed a little but not crushed to allow the steam to seep in.

Safety: At the end of the distillation process, the pot should be allowed to cool down before opening it for cleaning, to allow the pressure to drop and avoid splashing water and burning plants.

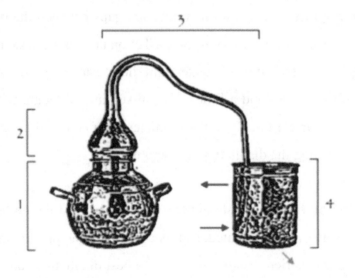

The different parts of the pot still: the pot that receives water and plant material (1), the lid (2), the swan neck (3), water pot containing the coil (4). The blue arrows indicate the correct direction of water flow. The ochre arrow indicates the place where the oil and floral water are collected.

Advantages and disadvantages: This alembic is the closest to what was done in the Middle Ages. Its main advantage is its simplicity of use and its rapidity of installation. However, its use has been progressively abandoned by professionals because of the direct contact between the plant material and the water, which can alter the quality of the distillation result. Indeed, some compounds tend to solubilise with the water in the still. Moreover, amateurs will be confronted with the absence of literature documenting precisely the volume of water in which to distil each plant, or what is the ideal volume of material to put in each still.

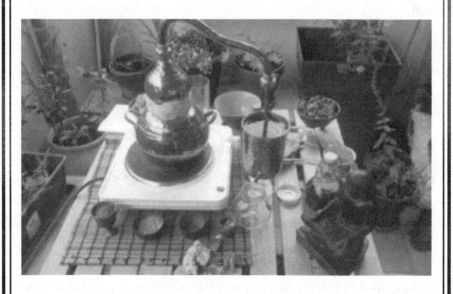

The still is heating up...

Column stills

Description and implementation: The column alembic differs from its potted cousin in that it has a high column where the plant material is placed. At the base of the column, a screen prevents the plants from falling into the water, while allowing the vapours to pass through. The material to be distilled must be placed densely in the column, while leaving enough space for the water vapour to circulate between the leaves and flowers.

Cooling: The cooling system is the same as for the traditional pot still.

Avoiding waste: Again, all joints of the parts will need to be sealed, often with Teflon tape or bread dough.

Duration of distillation: Distillation runs are often short. The oil production should be monitored on a case-by-case basis and distillation stopped when the still is no longer productive. It should be noted that the various sources report distillations that are often quite rapid, lasting half an hour or an hour. Sometimes, for certain leaves, notably Eucalyptus or Laurel, distillations are a little longer.

Proportions: The volume of water in the pot does not matter, but the various experiments found in the literature report better yields around 2 volumes of water compared to the same volume of plant material depending on whether you are distilling flower heads or leaves. Too much (or too little) water will result in a lower yield. Here again, there is no consensus on the optimal temperature and duration of distillation since this varies according to the equipment used, the volume of plant material, etc.

Safety: At the end of the distillation process, it is imperative to let the whole still cool down before opening it for cleaning.

Advantages and disadvantages: The advantage of this alembic is that it allows steam distillation without any contact between the hot water and the plant. Indeed, this contact can denature the oils. It also allows for finer control of the distillation temperature. Its disadvantages are obviously its greater volume and its higher cost.

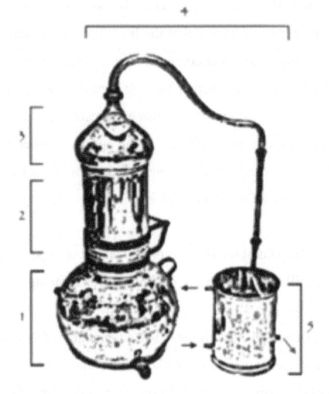

The different parts of the column still: the cucurbit that receives the water (1), the column that receives the plant material (2), the lid (3), the swan neck (4), the coil (5). The blue arrows indicate the correct direction of water flow. The ochre arrow indicates the place where the oil and floral water are collected.

- <u>Chemist's still</u>

Description and implementation: Made of glass, a chemist's alembic is made from a container, *the flask*, usually placed in a heating flask. On top of this flask is a distillation head (comparable to the head of a numbered still), followed by a water-cooled condenser (equivalent to a coil) and a receiver flask. Note the possibility of adding a Vigreux column on top of the flask, which allows fractional distillation and finer separation of the elements according to their volatility.

Advantages and disadvantages: Chemistry tools allow for more accurate distillations in controlled media. However, this method suffers from the same limitations as pot still distillation where the substrate is not separated from the water. In addition, the glassware is fragile and is often designed for very small volumes.

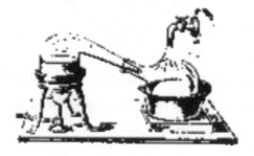

Distillation glassware.

Wok distillation

In ancient times, distillation was probably carried out using clay systems. This type of distillation, whose materials are quite accessible (clay, water, a baking skin), requires great technical rigour with no guarantee of results. As we have not succeeded in distilling oils with such a device, we will limit ourselves to describing it.

Description and implementation: a skin is stretched over a clay pot.

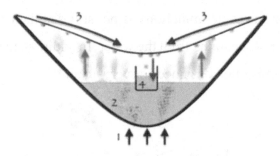

The heat source (1) causes the water and oils from the plant material placed in the clay pot (2) to evaporate. These condense on the skin and drip (3) until they drain into a cup placed in the centre of the device (4).

Advantages and disadvantages: This technique, known for the distillation of sea water, cannot in our opinion produce an essential oil or even a quality floral water. The mixture would be impure and contaminated by the clay in the container or the various substances used to treat the skin. The numerous leaks would lead to a low yield. Finally, the droplets could run off and fall back into the water, which would greatly degrade the quality of the final product. It is nevertheless useful for educational purposes...

A similar device can be made with a cooking-pot filled with the material you wish to distil, on top of which you place an upside-down pot lid (or wok) filled with water. In the centre of the pot, a small pot will be placed to collect the water that runs under the lid...

The steps are as follows:
Unscrew the handle on the lid and turn it to the other side (be careful not to overtighten it when turning it the other way, otherwise the glass may break). **Place the plant material in the water at the bottom of the pot**. Note that if you have two tiers of couscous pots, you can put the water at the bottom, then place the plant material in the first tier. For safety reasons, keep **volumes small** (up to a maximum of 1/4 of the filled pot).

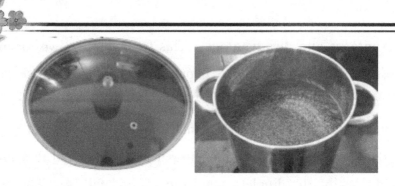

Place a couscoussier with a bowl in the centre on top. This is the bowl that will receive the vapours that have condensed on the lid. **Place the lid upside down on top of the assembly** (the handle points to the sky, and the lid is like a cup whose deepest point is just above the receiving bowl). You can plug the small safety cap on the lid, to prevent steam from escaping: beware as detailed below, this is not without risk!

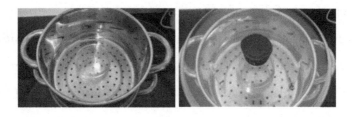

Put ice cubes on the lid. You will have to change the ice cubes and the water in the lid regularly, as the vapours will heat the glass and melt your ice cubes... You can imagine circuits with communicating vessels to drain the water but this is more complex. If this is too tedious, you can put a wok in place of the lid: it will contain more water and will heat up more slowly. However, you will not be able to monitor the progress of the distillation through the glass. It is also possible to make this device from a **steam juicer**.

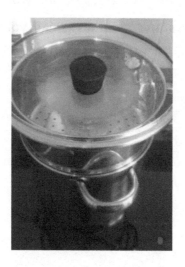

Note also that this device can give you oil for high-yielding plants (lavender, eucalyptus, rosemary, etc.). **However, don't expect too much from low yield plants**. The oil yield will often be derisory or even absent! In any case, you'll always get nice smelling hydrosol.

Caution: Like the pressure cooker still (described below), this device does not have a safety valve in case of excess pressure. There are many risks if the pressure rises too high: the glass in the lid can shatter, the pot and the couscous pot can come apart and cause boiling water to spurt out...

In practice, there will be leaks and it is unlikely that the device will explode under pressure. Nevertheless, you will have to **be careful about temperatures and volumes** (small volumes of water and plants). This handling is at your own risk!

- <u>Pressure cooker still</u>

It is possible to make distillation equipment using a pressure cooker.

Description and implementation: A copper pipe bent into a swan neck is fitted to the pressure valve of the cooker. It then passes through a tank of cold water before flowing into the collection container. The vegetable mixture can be placed in a couscous-type basket out of contact with the water in the cooker chamber.

Advantages and disadvantages: It goes without saying that such an arrangement can be dangerous (no control of pressure or temperature), with the risk of the boiling liquid spurting out and causing serious burns. In addition to being dangerous, the products distilled using such a set-up would not come close in quality to the essence extracted by a real steam still with elegant and useful shapes. Rather than tempting the devil, isn't it easier to order a small still that complies with local legislation on the web?

7. Distillation: Example of pot distillation

To start distilling, we advise you to **aim for high-yielding plants, such as lavender, eucalyptus, rosemary, and clove**, which give very satisfactory results. These plants (inexpensive and easily accessible) will allow you to get the hang of it. Let's look at an example of distillation, step by step.

First, **place the plants and water in the pot of your alembic**, then mount its lid on top.

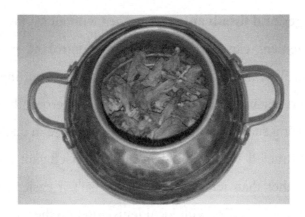

In a separate container, **make a small ball of dough** using flour mixed with a few spoonfuls of water and seal the various joints of the still with it.

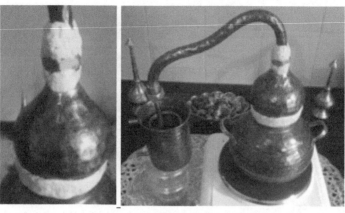

Screw a collar with a nipple (available at the hardware store) **onto a nearby sink spout** and **fit a plastic pipe** of suitable diameter (also available at the hardware store):

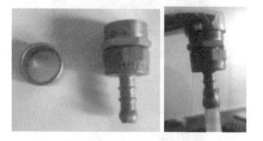

Fit the tube to the still, on the lowest copper inlet (pink arrow). Put another pipe (blue arrow) on top, for the water outlet. Open the tap and let a trickle of water flow slowly.

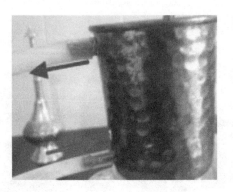

Place a flask or beaker under the mouth from which the oils will flow. You can now start the fire (electric hob or gas cooker), making sure to keep the heat low. The oil will start to flow after about 20 minutes.

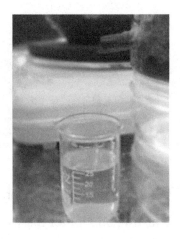

8. Distillation: Separating the oil from the hydrosol

It's done. The alembic is on the fire. A delicious smell fills the room, while drops gently trickle out of the copper pipe into your glass vial. It will not have escaped your attention that the liquid collected has an aqueous phase (the floral water) and a supernatant (the essential oil)[2] . Once distillation is complete, the aim is to separate the floral water from the oil. From this point on, everything depends on the volume of oil.

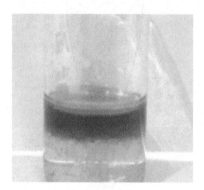

For large volumes, it is easiest to use a separating funnel, as illustrated below. Drop the distillation product into the separating funnel (1), wait a few tens of minutes for the phases to form, then

---

[2] Sometimes the oil is denser than the water, in which case it will be at the bottom. The density of each oil is specified in the next chapter.

purge the floral water into a container (2) using the tap. Only the oil will remain, which will be collected in another vial, ideally in opaque glass.

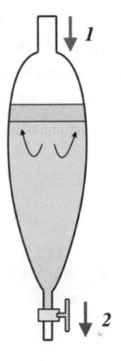

Decanting funnel used to separate two immiscible products: the oil phase (yellow) and the water phase (blue) using the tap.

As regards the choice of the decanting bulb, it is essential to choose a model made of chemical glass (borosilicate): PVC and plastics are not inert to certain compounds in oils and there is a high risk that you will find polymers dissolved in the oil (or worse: the oil will pierce your container if it stays there too long).

It is also important to choose a **decanting funnel at the right size for your distillation volume**. Oil droplets can settle on the surface of the glass, causing losses and reducing the yield of the distillation. The same applies to the still's outlet container. Therefore, avoid transferring the result of the distillation into several different containers.

The use of a decanter is therefore only recommended for large distillations with large stills. On small stills, the losses will be too great to make this method effective.

An alternative to the decanting funnel is to use an **essencier, such as the Florentine Flask.**

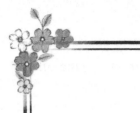

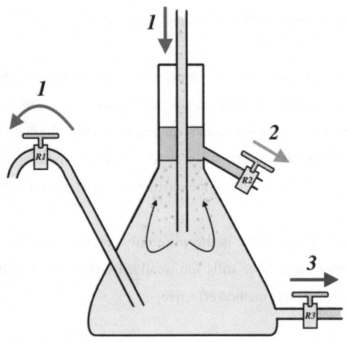

Essencier - Florentine vase allowing the separation of two
immiscible phases: the oil phase (yellow) and the water phase
(blue) by means of different taps.

The principle of the Florentine Flask is as follows:
1) During the distillation phase, valve R1 is open (it lets the liquid
flow), the others are closed.

2) The mixture of oil and floral water coming out of the still arrives through the pipe marked with the red arrow, and gradually fills the main flask.

3) By the principle of communicating vessels, the excess floral water will escape through the pipe marked by the pink arrow (R1). The oil, less dense than the water, will go to the surface (black arrows).

4) At the end of the distillation process, open tap R2 to collect the oil.

5) Then, to collect the remaining floral water, open the R3 tap.

This system is more efficient than the simple separating funnel and limits the loss of oil through deposits on the walls of the glassware. It is also more expensive.

Caution: unlike the separating funnel, it is ineffective in cases where the oil is denser than water.

For small volumes, the task will sometimes be disappointing and will (almost) always require great care. Using a syringe, carefully and directly extract the oil from the collection flask and transfer it to a separate flask. If a syringe is not available, there are glass dropper pipettes available on the market that will do the trick!

Whatever method you choose, don't forget to read the volume of oil collected, which will often be a few drops...

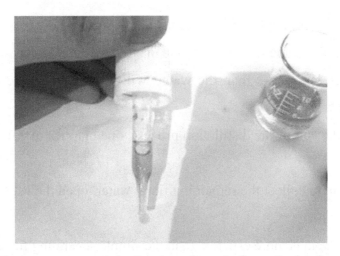

Rosemary essential oil, taken directly from the beaker.

Caution: do not empty the floral water from the container **before** the oil. If you do so, as the level of floral water drops, the oil will settle on the sides of the beaker, and you will end up with almost nothing.

If the oil is denser than the water (e.g. cinnamon, clove), we advise you to carefully remove the floral water that is floating on top of the oil. When there are only a few millilitres left (with the oil at the bottom), pour the whole (remaining floral water + oil) into a small beaker. You can then gently suck up the remaining floral water with a syringe to completely isolate the oil.

Use the floral water in the syringe to clean the bottom of the first container: there is often some oil trapped at the bottom!

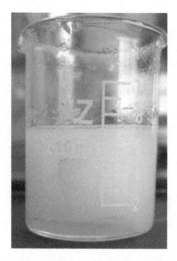

Cinnamon essential oil, denser than water

In industry, some laboratories use solvents that are miscible with the oil to separate it more easily from the water (the oil dissolves in the large volume of solvent, which is thus more easily separated from the water). They then separate the oil from the solvent by boiling the mixture: the solvent evaporates at a lower temperature than the oil, leaving only the oil at the end. This technique is often criticized because it is possible to find traces of the solvent, often toxic, in the final product. We do not recommend it.

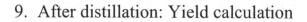

9. After distillation: Yield calculation

You can calculate the yield of your distillation using the following formula:

$$Yield = Volume\ of\ Oil\ /\ Plant\ Mass$$

It will allow you to measure the efficiency of your distillation method, to compare plants with each other, and to improve your technique.

We have detailed in the following chapters the expected yield for each plant. Note that the reported values differ greatly between sources, so they are only indicative. For example, in The Essential Oil Maker's Handbook[3] , which is a reference in the field, the yield of rosemary is 1 to 2%. Our experience with stems harvested in the woods has brought us closer to 5%!

---

[3] By Bettina Malle and Helge Schmickl, published by Spikehorn

10. After distillation: Conservation

The main environmental factors that degrade oils are light, humidity, oxygen, heat and time. Oxygen and humidity thicken essences by transforming them into resin (this is particularly true for lemon oils). Light alters the fragrance of most essences.

In fact, it is essential to store oils in a **tightly sealed, well-filled, opaque glass** environment and not to keep them for too long.

Storage in a plastic container is **not recommended,** as the oil can degrade the PVC of the wall and polymerise[4] . In general, there is no need to store oils in a cool place; storage at room temperature is usually sufficient.

It should be noted that even with these precautions the oils can degrade and molecular rearrangements with oxidation reactions of the various compounds occur. The shelf life of the various oils ranges from several months to several years. Although the ageing of oils is little studied, it is known, for example, that fennel oil

---

[4] In our experience, this even occurred during storage in medical biological sample tubes.

degrades in only two months. There is no general rule, but simply that oils should not be stored for longer than a few months.

The same packaging rules apply to hydrosols, except that they must be kept cool and are more rapidly perishable.

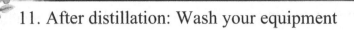

11. After distillation: Wash your equipment

Always wash your glassware thoroughly between distillations with **household alcohol**. Even after washing with soap and water and then with alcohol, oil droplets often remain on the walls of the containers. Do not hesitate to repeat the operation several times, as some odours (such as garlic) are extremely persistent.

To wash the copper still, a simple lemon is all that is needed: rub with a **sponge or soft cloth** and the copper will regain its shine! Do not use any potentially abrasive chemical product for this operation: it will attack the copper and you may find traces of it in your oils... Do not use a brush or steel wool either, which could scratch the copper. Store your still in the open air after drying it thoroughly. This will increase its life span.

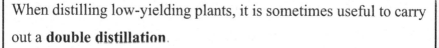

12. The case of low-yielding plants

When distilling low-yielding plants, it is sometimes useful to carry out a **double distillation**.

Double distillation consists of redistilling the hydrosol alone obtained at the end of a first distillation. It is possible to add fresh flowers to the hydrosol for this second distillation. This technique is mainly used for roses, to produce rose oil and rose water. Note that you must have recovered a significant volume of hydrosol: otherwise, there will not be enough oil to recover. We will detail the making of hydrosol in a dedicated chapter.

13. The case of fragile plants (Enfleurage)

Enfleurage is a scent extraction technique known since antiquity. It uses the property of fats to absorb the scents of the plants. In perfumery, there is hot enfleurage (or maceration) and cold enfleurage. Particularly adapted for plants with a soft or fragile fragrance, these demanding techniques allow to obtain rich perfumes.

Hot enfleurage: Throw the fresh flowers into a pot filled with animal fat. Heat it over low heat. Stir the mixture regularly with a wooden spatula until the fat is saturated with the smell. Leave to stand for a day, then repeat the operation as many times as necessary.

Next, filter the mixture and add one to two volumes of ethanol (the amount is up to you, depending on how saturated you want the scent to be). The addition of alcohol is called "washing" in perfumery. Shake vigorously for about ten minutes and then leave to stand. This will allow the ethanol to absorb the fragrances. Separate the ethanol from the fat with a coffee filter. Remove the plant debris from the fat. You can make perfume with the ethanol and ointments with the fat.

Tip: It is possible to do the same technique at room temperature, but over several days. If you heat the mixture, you can put the plant material in a tea filter with large enough pores. This will make the filtering easier.

This method is particularly suitable for flowers with discreet fragrances, such as orange blossom.

Cold enfleurage: This technique, which is much more rigorous, is used for jasmine, rose, violet or tuberose. This time, a little animal fat is applied to a glass panel in a layer of about one centimetre (the surface of fat to be applied will depend on the quantity of petals you have). Flower petals will be placed on the fat for one to three days, then removed and replaced with fresh flower petals. In this way, the fat will capture the discreet scents of the flower, without altering them by raising the temperature. This process should be repeated for several weeks until the fat is saturated with scent. One kilo of fat can absorb the scent of three kilos of flowers!

The panel should be kept cool. At the end of this period, collect the fat (dehairing), add alcohol (washing, about two parts alcohol to one part fat), then leave it again in a cool place for several weeks, stirring regularly. Finally, separate the fat from the alcohol using, for example, a coffee filter: here again you can make perfume and ointments.

Historically animal fat was animal (a 1/3 or 2/3 **pork fat/beef fat** mix for example). We recommend this mixture, although you can also get some results with a 70%/30% Vaseline/Glycerine mixture in case you can't get any fat. Beware, the mixture with Vaseline is much less efficient than fat: Vaseline has a much lower absorbency and is somewhat soluble with alcohol.

Here is an example of a cold enfleurage: Get two small picture frames with glass panels. Take the glass panel from the 2nd frame and put it aside for now.

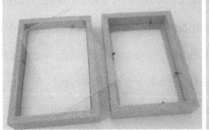 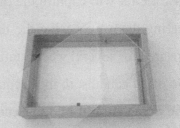

Pull up the tabs under the frame you will be using. The second glass panel will be placed on top!

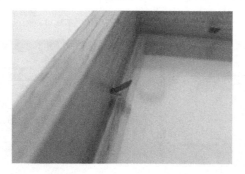

Mix 70g of lard with 30g of beef fat in a glass jar. Shake the mixture well.

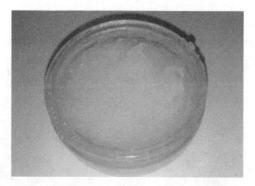

Place half of the mixture you have just made on the back of the glass panel of the photo frame. Carefully place the petals in it and put some fat back on top of the petals.

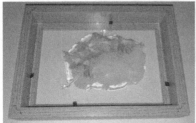
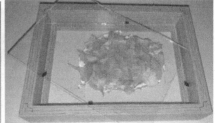

Place the second glass panel at the back, so that the flowers and fat are squashed between the glass panels. Your enfleurage frame is ready. Leave it to rest in a cool place.

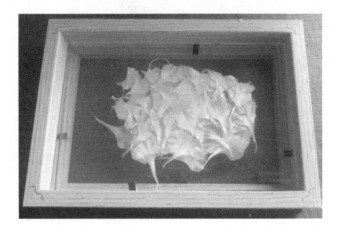

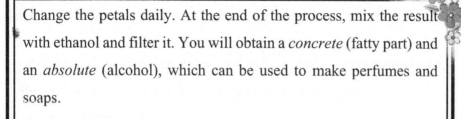

Change the petals daily. At the end of the process, mix the result with ethanol and filter it. You will obtain a *concrete* (fatty part) and an *absolute* (alcohol), which can be used to make perfumes and soaps.

14. The case of cold pressing

Cold pressing is a gentle technique for extracting oil from a number of plants, such as the olive. The term 'extra virgin' on olive oil means that your oil is the product of a single cold pressing of the olives. In 'only' virgin oils, manufacturers sometimes press the olives a second time to maximise their yield, which can increase the acidity of the oil and alter its taste. Cold pressing can also be used to extract oil from lemon, orange, or bergamot peel for example.

The technical procedure, although simple, can be a real challenge for the ill-equipped individual. Of course, you can try to crush the peeled peel by hand with a spatula, for example, but this will take a long time and the result will be rather disappointing. The easiest way to do this is to buy a mechanical press mounted on a worm gear, as shown below. The material to be pressed is placed in the tank (1), while the auger (2) presses the mixture that is collected at the outlet. The mixture should be left to stand for several days to allow the oil to separate from the water phase. You can then filter the product and separate it in a separating funnel to isolate the oil.

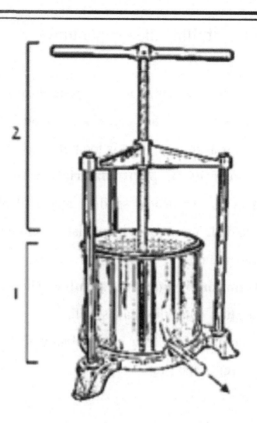

Cold press: the product will have to rest for several days so that the aqueous and oily phases separate.

15. Tip: Controlling the temperature

Temperature control is essential for successful distillation. Neither too cold nor too hot. Distillations are done around 100°. There are several indications as to whether it is too hot or too cold:

- If you see deposits of plant material at the end of the distillation process, the heat is sending pieces of plant material directly into the coil. You should immediately remove the fire and *reduce* the temperature.

- If you see steam coming out of the alembic (where the oil should be coming out), turn *down* the heat as well.

- If nothing comes out... you are probably too cold. Slowly *increase* the power of the fire.

If you do not have a thermometer on your still to check the internal temperature, there is a simple way to find out the approximate temperature of the water. Put a drop of water on the copper surface of the still and count how many seconds it takes to evaporate.

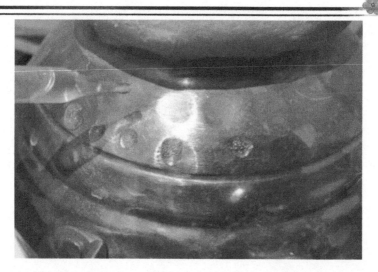

A few drops are delicately placed on the still...

The chart below gives an idea of the survival time of the drop as a function of temperature on a metal wall. Note that the values in the table are approximate to within one or two seconds. The survival time of the water changes according to the type of metal in the still (different heat transfer capacity).

Overall, the drop should last between 15 and 25 seconds. If it evaporates in less than 10 seconds, you are above 130°C (which is too hot for distillation).

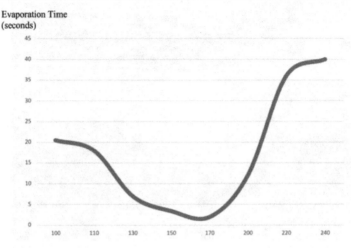

Evaporation Time (seconds)

Temperature (°C)

Note that above a certain temperature (180°C), the survival time of the water drop increases: this is due to the Leidenfrost effect. The surface is so hot that a film of vapour forms under the drop and causes it to bounce off (like on a hot stove).

This technique will not give you the temperature to the nearest degree... but it can be very useful!

16. Tip: Save water

On your first few distillations, you will be amazed at how much water is wasted. Even with a small trickle of water to cool the coil, a one-hour distillation can easily consume 20-30 litres of water. This is a lot of water. One way to save water is to get a small submersible electric sprinkler pump and set up a closed water circuit.

We advise you to take a model that works with 5V. This can be easily found by searching for **"5V DC USB water pump"** in the various search engines. Such a pump costs a maximum of about 20 euros.

Some models can be plugged directly into a USB socket (hence the 5 volts, nominal voltage of a USB port): this is the easiest way! This will avoid having to solder wires with an external battery, or having to change the batteries regularly...

WARNING: Connect the motor plugs to a USB socket (but not to the USB plug of your computer... In which case it is probably microprocessor hydrosol that you will get back...)

Once you have your motor in hand, fit the hoses to your still and place it in the bottom of a water tank. The water tank should hold at least 10 litres, so that it does not heat up too quickly. You can also put some ice packs in the tray. You can reuse this water during your distillations. You can also use it to water plants afterwards, etc.

Depending on the diameter of your pipes, it may happen that the **motor pumps too hard** and causes the water to overflow into the still's cooling tank... If this happens there are two solutions:

- Elevate your still in relation to the water pan (e.g. by placing the water pan on the floor and the still on a table). The water flow will decrease.

- Extend the distance of the hose from the motor to the inlet of the still. As the length increases, the resistance to water flow will also increase and the flow rate will decrease.

If you are a handyman: you can also mount a resistor in series on one of the motor plugs to reduce the current flowing through the motor. Make sure you size your resistor properly if you do this: the motor consumes around 200 or 300mA, at 5V, it tends to heat up quickly...

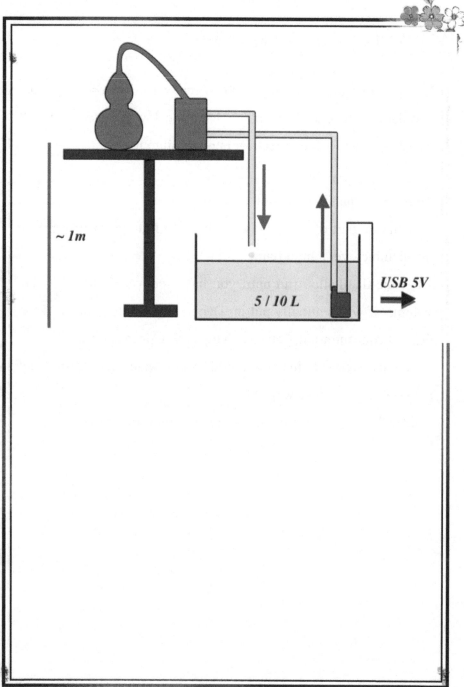

~ 1m

5 / 10 L

USB 5V

17. Tip: distilling floral water

It is possible that you only want to recover a hydrosol from the distillation process. Some plants have too low a yield, so it will simply be impossible to recover enough oil to use it.

To obtain a quality hydrosol:

- Distil one part of the plant with **three to four parts** of water in the alembic over a high flame.
- Let the distillation run until you have recovered half (1/2) the volume of water initially put in. Depending on the plants and the desired concentration, you can change these proportions.
- You can redistil this water with fresh water and fresh plant material (e.g. for rose water).
- Filter the mixture in case there are still impurities in it.

IV - Plants and their uses

In this section, we will detail for a set of plants the main information needed from harvesting to distillation.

The values given (density, yield, flash point, molecule content, etc.) are indicative: they correspond to values commonly found in the literature. There will **always be** a difference in relation to the properties of the plants you distil, as explained in the chapter on the variability factors of oils.

Anise: (Star and Green Anise)

Illicium Verum - Pimpinella Anisum

Native to Asia, star anise (Chinese star anise) is more aromatic than its European cousin, green anise.

Plant material: Star anise or green anise seeds. The seeds are harvested in autumn when the plant is mature. Caution: its cousin the Japanese star anise is toxic. The seeds are harvested from August to September.

Example of recipe: Gently crush the seeds with a mortar and pestle, then steam distil one unit of aniseed into one and a half units of water.

Oil yield	Flashpoint	Density at 25°C
1 to 5% (Star A.) 2 to 3.5% (Green A.)	93°C (Star A.) 101°C (Green A.)	0.97
Contains:	Anethol, Shikimic acid	

Product: Colourless or pale-yellow essential oil with a characteristic aniseed odour, floral water.

Popular virtues:

- Antispasmodic
- Carminative
- Relaxing, promotes sleep

Good to know: Anise was brought to Europe in the late Middle Ages by none other than the Venetian explorer Marco Polo. It was one of the most valuable spices in the West at the time.

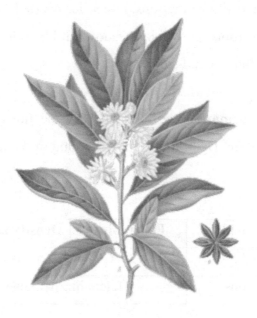

Arnica

Arnica montana

Arnica is a family of wild, mountainous plants known for treating bruises and contusions.

Precautions: Do not apply to open wounds, irritant.

Plant material: Flowering tops. Green leaves (before flowering) and fermented roots. Grows in meadows at high altitudes (above 800m), from June to mid-July.

Example of recipe: Harvest, cut and dry the flowering tops at room temperature. Distil for 30 minutes 300g of Arnica in 300mL of water.

Oil yield	Flashpoint	Density at 25°C
0.1 à 0.3%	> 130°C	0.9
Contains:	Helenalin, Arnicine	

Product: Yellow to brown essential oil with a discreet odour, floral water.

Popular virtues:

- Analgesic, used against the pain of contusions, bruises, stings
- Anti-inflammatory
- Antirheumatic

Cream for bruises: Leave 200g of fresh flowers (or 600g of dried flowers) to macerate for 4 weeks in 50mL of vegetable oil in a bowl sterilised in boiling water. Filter and put in an opaque bottle. Store in a cool place. It is possible to add a few drops of Italian Helichrysum oil, a healing agent, and beeswax.

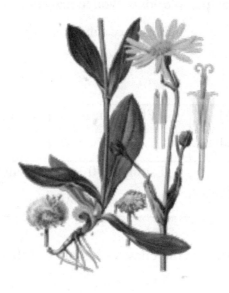

Basil

Ocimum Basilicum

A fragrant plant with many virtues, it repels insect pests of crops. There are more than 60 varieties.

Plant material: Leaves, flowers, or whole plant. The vegetative season (April to October) is the best time for harvesting. Distillation must be rapid. The yield is very low.

Example of a recipe: We advise you to macerate in a base of olive oil for example... The yield is very small and will almost always be disappointing.

Oil yield	Flashpoint	Density at 25°C
0.02 à 0.04%	80°C	0.9
Contains:	Estragol (70-80%), Linalool (1 to 30%)	

Product: A few drops of yellow essential oil with a basilica smell.

Popular virtues:

- Antispasmodic
- Anti-infective
- Calming
- Relaxing

Good to know: Basil, the "royal plant", was only served at the table of the Roman emperors. It was also used for mummification, probably for its antibacterial properties.

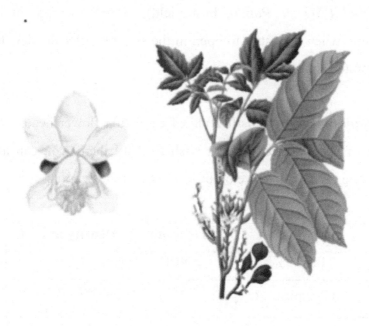

Calendula officinalis

Calendula officinalis

Also known as marigolds, its flowers close at night and open when the sun is high in the sky. It blooms in spring. Its flowers are edible.

Plant material: Flowers and stems of *Calendula Officinalis* or marigold (*Tagetes Patula*, best yield), after flowering, in the morning when they start to open in the sun, but after the dew has evaporated.

Example of recipe: Distil 200g of calendula flower heads with 250g of water. If you do not wish to distil them, you can also macerate them in an olive oil base to extract the benefits.

Oil yield	Flashpoint	Density at 25°C
0.1 à 0.5%	>90°C	0.9
Contains:	Carotenoids, Salicylic acid, Alcohols, α-Thuene (25%)	

Product: Red-yellow to amber coloured oil.

Popular virtues:

- Analgesics
- Antiseptics
- Relieves cramps

Please note: Please note that hybrids and new decorative varieties contain very little oil.

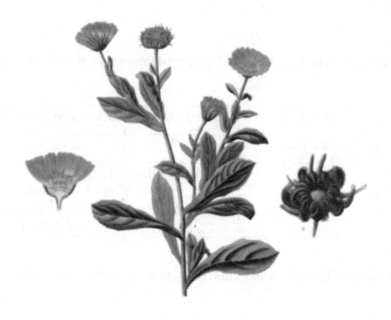

Cardamom

Elettaria cardamomum

Originally from South-East Asia, cardamom can be cultivated (on a veranda) in our latitudes.

Plant material: Seed only, present in harvested fruit when the plant is more than two years old.

Example of recipe: Distil 200g of cardamom into 300mL of water.

Oil yield	Flashpoint	Density at 25°C
4 - 7%	57°C	0.92
Contains:	Terpinyl acetate (<45%), 1-8-Cineole (<33%), Limonene, Linalool, α-Terpineole, Myrcene, α-Pinene, Citral, Geraniol (<2%)	

Product: Pale yellow essential oil with a characteristic spicy smell.

Popular virtues:

- Improves mood
- Beneficial for digestion

Good to know: Cardamom has many virtues, including that of reducing the effects of caffeine by catalysing its elimination. It also reduces the smell of garlic after ingestion.

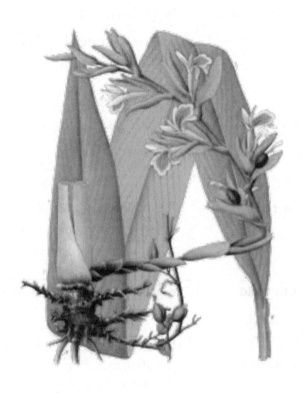

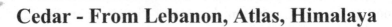

Cedar - From Lebanon, Atlas, Himalaya

Cedrus - Libani, Atlantica, Deodara

Many varieties of trees are falsely called cedar and are not related to the genus *Cedrus*. Their species are often highly toxic (*Red Cedar, Thuja, White Cedar...*)

Plant material: Bark chopped into fine pieces. It is possible to distil the leaves, but for a lower yield.

Example of recipe: Distil 200g of finely ground cedar bark into 400mL of water.

Oil yield	Flashpoint	Density at 25°C
2 à 5%	93°C	0.9
Contains:	Himachalene (α, β, and γ, 70%), a-Atlantone (5%), Gatlantone (5%), Himachol (4%)	

Product: Pale yellow to brown oil, with a woody, sweet smell.

Popular virtues:
- Antiseptic

- Antifungal
- Anti-inflammatory
- Reduces stress

Good to know: Cedar wood has been used since ancient times by the ancient Egyptians and Assyrians as a shield against demons and diseases...

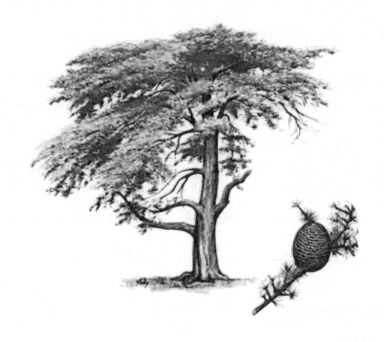

Celery

Apium graveolens

Plant material: The whole plant can be distilled, but the essential oils are found in the seeds. Harvesting takes place in late summer (September/October).

Example of recipe: Gently crush the seeds and distil them into one and a half cups of water.

Oil yield	Flashpoint	Density at 25°C
3% (seeds) 0.1% (leaves)	>65°C	0.8
Contains:	D-Limonene (50 to 75%), Myrcene (1 to 5%), β-pinene (<1%)	

Product: Brown essential oil with a characteristic smell.

Popular virtues:

- Toning
- Stomachic
- Diuretic

- Aphrodisiac

Good to know: The first traces of celery use date back to the ancient Greeks.

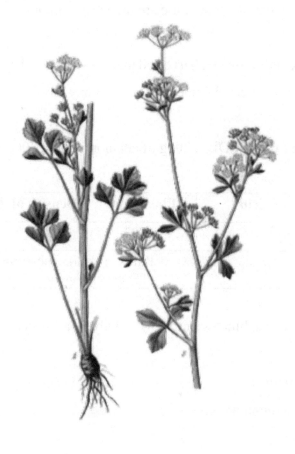

Chamomile

Anthemis Nobilis, Latriarca Chamomilla

There are several varieties of chamomile, Roman chamomile and German chamomile are the most common.

Plant material: Flowers, harvested in the morning at the beginning of the flowering period (June) on a very sunny day.

Example of recipe: Distil 200g of chamomile into 300g of water.

Oil yield	Flashpoint	Density at 25°C
0.1 à 1%	50°C	0.9
Contains:	α-Pinene (15%), Eucalyptol (15%), Limonene (5%)	

Product: Intense blue essential oil, cloudy floral water.

Popular virtues:

- Anti-inflammatory
- Relaxing
- Antirheumatic

Good to know: Chamomile can be very easily sown in a garden and will tend to spread spontaneously wherever it finds space. You can then grow your own crop.

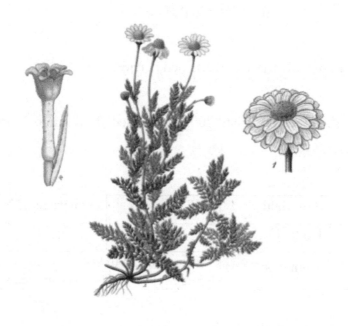

Chilli

Pimenta officinalis

There are various colours of chilli pepper. Each one designates the fruit of a different species.

Plant material: Dried and crushed berries.

Example of recipe: Distil 200g of crushed chillies into 300mL of water.

Oil yield	Flashpoint	Density at 25°C
Up to 4%.	93°C	1.04
Contains:	Eugenol (50 to 90%), Methyl-Eugenol (1 to 5%), Terpinolene	

Product: Essential oils denser than water, yellow or amber in colour, with a characteristic chilli smell.

Popular virtues:
- Anti-inflammatory
- Anti-infective
- Antioxidant

- Analgesic

Good to know: In medical practice, hot pepper-based poultices (capsaicin) are used to treat intractable pain. The effectiveness of this molecule has been shown for neuropathic pain (nerve pain), but also in the context of osteoarthritis.

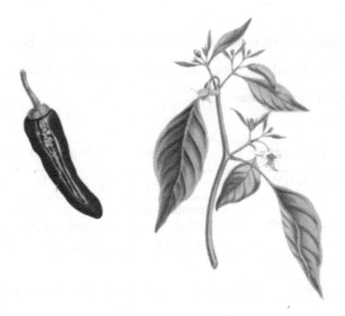

Cinnamon

Cinnamomum Zeylanicum

The tree is native to Sri Lanka and is cultivated in tropical regions. Cinnamon is made from its inner bark.

Plant material: Dried bark, branches, leaves and flowers.

Example of recipe: Crush 200g of dried cinnamon bark. Distil gently in 300mL of water. Be patient: the oil will settle at the bottom of the container.

Oil yield	Flashpoint	Density at 25°C
0.5 à 1.5%	92°C	1.05
Contains:	Cinnamaldehyde (50-75%), Eugenol (<5%), β-Caryophyllene (<2%), Linalool (<5%), Coumarin (<2%)	

Product: Pale to dark yellow essential oil with a higher density than the velvety white hydrosol.

Popular virtues:
- Antiseptic

- Stimulates circulation

Good to know: The quality of the original material is essential for a good yield. The floral water will have a white colour due to its high concentration of Cinnamaldehyde. Caution: Cinnamaldehyde can be toxic in large quantities. It is used both as a flavouring agent, in perfumery ... but as a fungicide in agriculture.

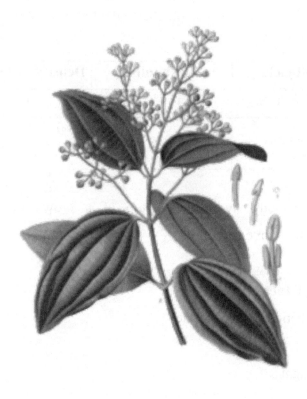

Clove

Syzygium aromaticum

Originating from an oceanic island, the clove tree has been known in Europe since antiquity.

Plant material: Clove, which will have been macerated for two to three days in water. You can practice a double distillation.

Oil yield	Flashpoint	Density at 25°C
15 à 20%	110°C	1.1
Contains:	Eugenol (75%) β-Caryophyllene (17%)	

Product: Cloudy hydrosol, on top of a brown oil with a characteristic clove smell.

Popular virtues:
- Anaesthetic (dental, muscle)
- Antibacterial
- Antifungal

Note: To test the oil content of the clove, you can put it in water: a clove with a high oil content will sink or stay upside down, while poor quality clove will float horizontally...

It is possible to separate the Eugenol from the rest of the oil by putting the oil in a 10% solution of potassium hydroxide: Eugenol will precipitate to the bottom and can be recovered.

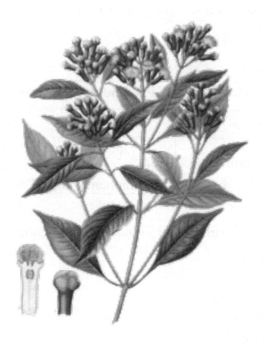

Coriander

Coriandrum sativum

Very present in our kitchens, coriander also has many medicinal virtues

Plant material: Seeds, stems and leaves, harvested between late July and September

Oil yield	Flashpoint	Density at 25°C
0.1 à 2%	62°C	0.8
Contains:	α-Pinene (70%), Camphene, β-pinene, Myrcene, Para-cymene, Limonene, and γ-Terpinene	

Product: Pale yellow or colourless essential oil with a characteristic odour.

Popular virtues:
- Antibacterial
- Antioxidant
- Promotes sleep

Good to know: Prolonging the distillation process will diminish the antioxidant capacities of coriander essential oil

(For more information, see [5])

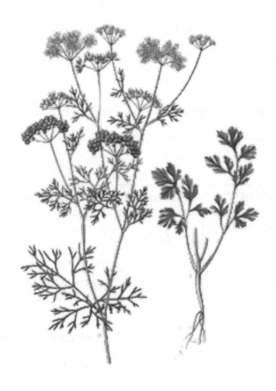

---

[5] *Hydrodistillation Extraction Time Effect on Essential Oil Yield, Composition, and Bioactivity of Coriander Oil* - Zheljazkov et. al,

Dill

Anethum graveolens

Plant material: The whole plant can be distilled, but the main part of the oil is in the seeds, to be harvested in early autumn. The leaves should be harvested before flowering (June to October).

Example of recipe: Distil the seeds and gently crush them in double the volume of water.

Oil yield	Flashpoint	Density at 25°C
2 to 4% (seeds) 0.2% (leaves)	60°C	0.9
Contains:	Anethol, Carvone, Tannins	

Product: Pale yellow essential oil supernatant on top of the hydrosol. Sweet, minty, herbaceous and fresh smell.

Popular virtues:
- Carminative: promotes the expulsion of intestinal gas
- Antispasmodic
- Sedative and analgesic
- Antimicrobial and antiparasitic

Good to know: Dill has been used in pharmacopoeia since ancient times. *Carvone, a molecule extracted from the essential oil of dill, is used as an anti-germinant on industrial potatoes.*

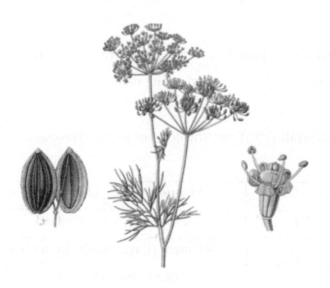

Eucalyptus (family)

Eucalyptus Globulus

Eucalyptus trees grow perfectly in our latitudes, and you can grow them on a sunny terrace.

Cautions: Eucalyptus leaves are highly **toxic.** If you are not a Koala, it is best to refrain from eating them...

Plant material: Dried and crushed Eucalyptus leaves.

Oil yield	Flashpoint	Density at 25°C
3 à 4%	49°C	0.91
Contains:	1-8 Cineol (Eucalyptol): from 60 to 85% depending on the species	

Product: Pale yellow essential oil.

Popular virtues:

- Respiratory comfort, cough relief
- Air freshener
- Analgesic

- Anti-inflammatory

Good to know: A single teaspoon of concentrated oil can kill a man. The distillation of Eucalyptus is very satisfactory with a good yield. Ideal for beginners.

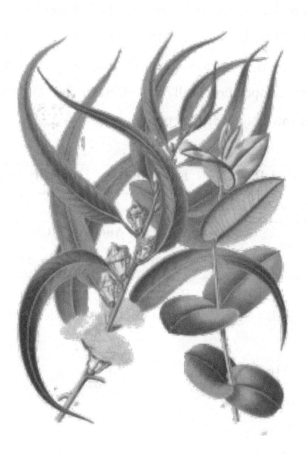

(Common) Fennel

Foeniculum vulgare

Fennel is a perennial, biennial plant, easily cultivated

Plant material: Seeds. To be harvested when their colour starts to turn brown, between August and October. It is also possible to distil the aerial parts, harvested between July and August, but the molecular composition will be different (up to 90% Trans-Anethole and up to 20% Fenchone).

Oil yield	Flashpoint	Density at 25°C
Up to 6%.	60°C	0.9
Contains:	Trans-Anethole (70%), Estragol (10%), Limonene (5%)	

Product: Yellow-green essential oil with a characteristic smell.

Popular virtues:

- Carminative
- Diuretic
- Antispasmodic

- Pest control

Good to know: In Rome, a crown of fennel was awarded to the most deserving gladiators in the arena...

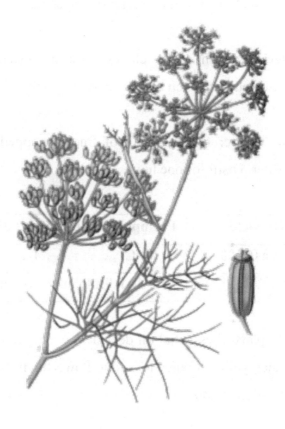

Garlic

Allium Sativum

Garlic belongs to the alliaceae family, along with onions and shallots. It is a powerful disinfectant.

Plant material: Fresh garlic cloves, best harvested between August and September, when the leaves start to wilt.

Example of recipe: Distil 400mg of finely chopped garlic in 600mL of water. Distil for one hour.

Oil yield	Flashpoint	Density at 25°C
0.1 à 0.4 %	53°C	1.1
Contains:	Allyl disulphide - Allicin	

Product: Droplets of essential oil deposited mainly at the bottom of the container, yellow-orange in colour. Powerful, persistent, and characteristic garlic odour.

Popular virtues:
- Reduction of arteriosclerosis

- Reduction of blood pressure
- Anti-inflammatory and antioxidant
- Disinfectant

Good to know: Allicin is the molecule responsible for the smell and taste of garlic. It has important antibiotic and antifungal properties. Highly volatile, it is synthesised and released when a garlic clove is injured, allowing the plant to protect itself. [6]

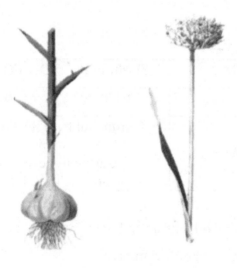

---

[6] Khan et al - Optimization of extraction of Garlic Essential Oil - 2017

Geranium (Pelargonium)

Pelargonium graveolens

Warning: The Rose Geranium, *often mistakenly called Geranium,* is the African cousin of the Pelargonium.

Plant material: Leaves and petals during flowering in spring. Most of the oil is in the young leaves. The stems are detrimental to the distillation process. Dry, the yield is lower but the quality higher.

Oil yield	Flashpoint	Density at 25°C
Up to 1%.	64°C	0.88
Contains:	Citronellol (<37%), Geranial (<25%), Linalool (<11%), β-Caryophyllene (<5%), Menthone, Citral, Limonene	

Product: Essential oil with an amber to greenish yellow colour and a pinkish odour, more or less minty.

Popular virtues:

- Liver detoxifier
- Analgesic

- Antiseptic

Good to know: The flowers and leaves **of the Rose Geranium** (and members of its family) contain almost no oil (unlike the **Pelargoniums**). Care should be taken not to make a mistake when buying or harvesting. The two plants are distinguished by the size of the flowers (smaller for the Geranium), as well as the hairs on the leaves of the Pelargoniums.

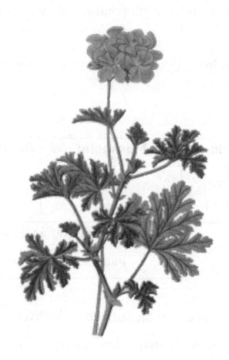

Ginger

Zingiber officinale

Native to India or China, ginger is a rhizome (root formation) with many virtues. However, few people know what the whole plant looks like.

Plant material: Roots and rhizome to maximise yield, fresh or dried. The roots should be chopped as finely as possible.

Example of recipe: 200g of very finely chopped ginger, in 300mL of water.

Oil yield	Flashpoint	Density at 25°C
2% (dry) 0.3% (fee)	57°C	0.87
Contains:	Zingiberene (60%), Eucalyptol, Farnesene, Curcumene,	

Product: Essential oil on the surface of the hydrosol with a yellow opalescent to yellow-brown colour and a strong, warm and spicy smell.

Popular virtues:

- Aphrodisiac
- Stimulates the appetite

Good to know: The word ginger derives from the Sanskrit *'srngavera'*: the shape of a deer's antler. Arab traders imported it along with slaves from the African horn, which gave the city of Zanzibar its name.

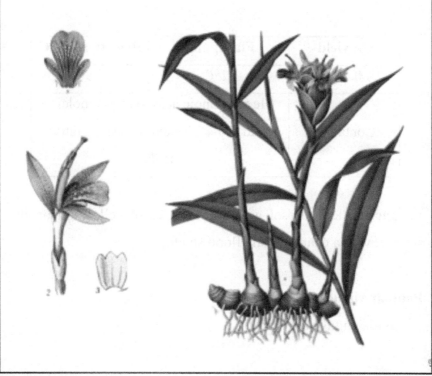

Hibiscus Althea

Hibiscus Syriacus

A genus of plants known since ancient times for their edible fruits, there are several hundred different types of hibiscuses

Plant material: Dried leaves and flower, seed (cold pressed)

Example of recipe: Distil 200g of dried and cut flowers in 300mL of water. Keep the bottom of the pot.

Oil yield	Flashpoint	Density at 25°C
0.1%	81°C	0.98
Contains:	Hexadecanoic acid (64%), Linoleic acid (20%), Linalool, various fatty acids	

Product: Pale hydrosol with a few tastes of yellow oil on the surface, with a characteristic floral smell.

Popular virtues:
- Nourishing for the skin

- Moisturizer
- Fight against skin ageing (vitamin E)

Hibiscus dye and ink:

Once the distillation of *Hibiscus Syriacus* is complete, collect the floral material and the red watery paste at the bottom. Leave it to macerate in a cool place for a few days in a base of water, then filter the mixture. You will obtain a thick red water loaded with Anthocyanin, a powerful colouring agent which gives the plant its colour. Can also be used as an ink and aroma. Keep the mixture in a cool place.

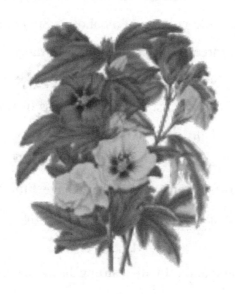

Jasmine from Spain

Jasminum Grandiflorum

In Persian, the term *Yasmine* means *divine gift* or *fragrant flower*.
Several dozen varieties exist.

Plant material: Flower heads, as soon as the bud has opened and the flower is fully open. Harvesting is done at dawn, after the first sun exposure, with immediate treatment of the flowers

Example of a recipe: Place the flowers in vegetable fat for *three* successive *weeks,* changing them *every 48 hours.* At the end, mix the fat with a double volume of alcohol (> 80°) in a jar, and let it rest for another three weeks, shaking the jar daily. When finished, filter the result: the alcohol can be used to make perfume, the fat for soap. The utensils must be made of glass or wood. Metal and plastic are forbidden.

Yield: 0.1%. Flash point and density have little meaning here, depending on the products used during enfleurage.

Product: Alcohol and oil with a strong Jasmine smell.

Popular virtues:

- Calming, soothing,
- Anxiolytic and sedative

Please note: The alcohol in the above recipe can be used directly as a perfume. It is possible to add a few drops of the oils of your choice, according to your imagination (e.g. rose). **As jasmine flagrance is altered by heat, distillation is prohibited.**

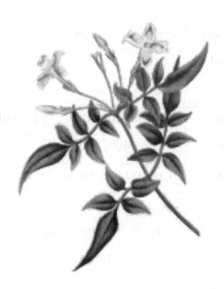

Laurel Tree

Laurus Nobilis

The leaves and flowers of the True Laurel are used in cooking as an aromatic.

Cautions: Not to be confused with oleander, which is fatally toxic.

Plant material: fruits, leaves, and twigs

Example of recipe: 200g of laurel leaves, ideally finely chopped, in 400mL of water.

Oil yield	Flashpoint	Density at 25°C
0.8 à 1.5%	49°C	0.9
Contains:	Eucalyptol (30%), Terpinyl, Linalool	

Product: Translucent floral water. Pale yellow surface oil with a penetrating, strong, spicy and camphorated odour.

Popular virtues:
- Antibacterial, anti-fungal

- Mucolytic, expectorant

Good to know: In France, the bay laurel was used in the Middle Ages to honour young doctors. It was called the *Bacca-Laurea* crown... Nowadays, the "Bacca-Laurea" is the French high school diploma.

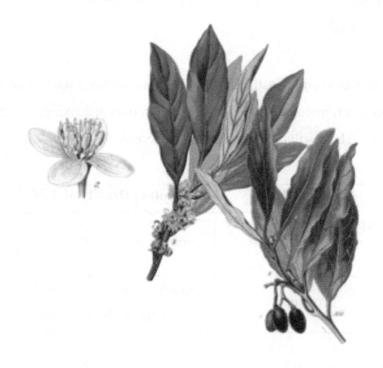

Lavender, Lavandin

Lavandula officinalis, Lavandula x intermedia

Of these fragrant plants used since Roman times to perfume clothes and spaces, lavandin has the highest oil yield.

Plant material: Flower tops or herbs, harvested around mid-August in full sun.

Example of recipe: Distil one volume of previously dried lavender flower heads in double the volume of water, over approximately 45 minutes. The distillation is quick and generous.

Oil yield	Flashpoint	Density at 25°C
Depending on the variety: Grass: 0.5 to 1.5%. Flowers: up to 5%.	> 60°C	0.8
Contains:	Linalool, Linalyl acetate, and Camphor (for Lavandin)	

Product: Pale yellow essential oil on the surface of the hydrosol. Intense scent of lavender.

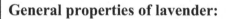

General properties of lavender:

- Calming,
- Healing, antiseptic and anti-venomous
- Antiseptic and bactericide

Good to know: In French, the word *Lavande comes* from the Latin *lavandaria:* the laundry to be washed. Lavandin can be distinguished by its two floral branches on the same stem and its powerful fragrance.

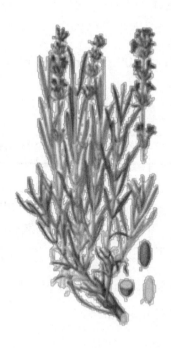

Lemon balm

Melissa officinalis

Lemon balm is an aromatic plant that has been used in pharmacopoeia since the Middle Ages. Be careful not to confuse its precious and expensive oil with counterfeits cut from lemongrass.

Plant material: fresh leaves harvested before flowering, in full sun and immediately distilled.

Example of recipe: Distil 200g of fresh plant material into 300g of water.

Oil yield	Flashpoint	Density at 25°C
Around 0.5%.	80°C	0.9
Contains:	β-pinene, Sabinene, E-Caryophyllene	

Product: Yellow or pale green droplets of oil supernatant on top of a hydrosol. Lemon balm odour.

Popular virtues:

- Antiviral
- Digestive (antispasmodic)
- Soothing and relaxing

Good to know: One of the first written references to Melissa dates to ancient Greece where *Theophrastus* called it a "bee plant" due to their great affinity for its nectar.

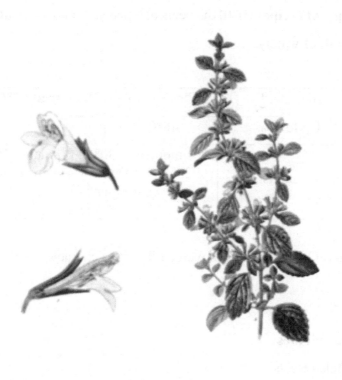

Lemongrass, Lemon

Citrus medica

Plant material: Pericarp (peel) of the lemon.

Preparation: As for the oranges, peel the lemons with a peeler, then chop the peel in a blender.

Example of recipe: Distil the peels of 8 peeled lemons (about 200g in 200mL of water).

Oil yield	Flashpoint	Density at 25°C
Up to 2%.	48°C	0.8
Contains:	D-limonene (>30%), β-pinene (10 to 20%), p-mentha-1,4-diene (5 to 10%), α-pinene (1 to 5%), Myrcene, Geranial.	

Product: Green to yellow covered oils with a characteristic lemony smell.

Popular virtues:

- Repels insects
- Analgesic

- Stimulates the appetite

Note: The oil can also be cold extracted, but its molecular composition will be different. It may cause more reactions when applied to the skin, especially in the sun. It is also common for a wax to be put on the lemon for preservation purposes. Wash and rub the lemons vigorously before distillation.

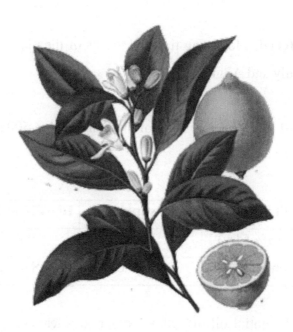

Marjolaine

Origanum majorana

Marjoram is the wild cousin of oregano. An annual perennial, it can easily be grown on a balcony for distillation...

Precautions: Contains various allergens

Plant material: Flowering tips and leaves of the plant, harvested between July and August.

Example of recipe: Distil 300g of plant material in 500g of water, at 100°C.

Oil yield	Flashpoint	Density at 25°C
0.7 to 1% (dry)	59°C	0.89
Contains:	Terpinenes, Thujanol, Sabinene	

Product: Essential oil of yellow colour (dry leaves) or greenish (fresh) on the surface of the Hydrosol. Aggressive odour similar to that of thyme.

Popular virtues:

- Relieves stress and anxiety
- Regulates sleep disorders
- Analgesic

Good to know: The goddess Aphrodite herself is said to have given the plant its scent. On their wedding day, Roman women wore a floral crown of marjoram and verbena.

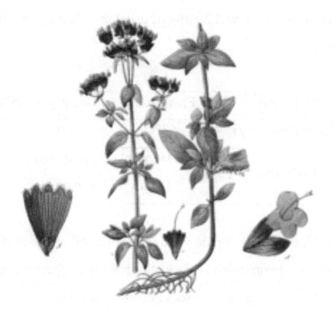

Mint - Peppermint

Mentha Spicata - Mentha x Piperita

Peppermint is the result of spontaneous hybridization between two types of mint and contains the highest levels of menthol.

Plant material: Leaves and flower heads of peppermint or spearmint. Spearmint oil is low in menthol but high in Carvone.

Example of recipe: Distil 200mg of dried mint leaves into 300mL of water.

Oil yield	Flashpoint	Density at 25°C
0.5 to 1.5% (dry)	62°C	0.88
Contains:	Menthol (Peppermint), Eucalyptol, Limonene	

Product: Transparent or pale yellow essential oil on the surface of the hydrosol. Characteristic minty odour. Only peppermint has the power and refreshing smell associated with menthol.

Popular virtues:

- Mucolytic
- Skin healing
- Calming

Good to know: Spearmint can be distinguished from peppermint by its light-coloured leaves, the absence of a stalk at the base of the leaves, and its sweet smell.

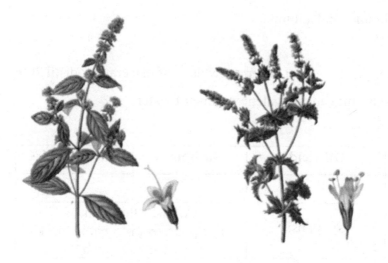

Pepper Mint   Common Mint

Mustard: white, field

Sinapis alba, Sinapis arvencis

Precautions: Brown mustard (Sinapis juncea) **and black mustard** contain **neurotoxic** elements (toxic for the neurons).

Plant material: Mustard seeds. These must have undergone a maceration phase in an equivalent volume of water for several days before being distilled. Harvesting is done when the pods start to dry in summer and autumn.

Example of recipe: After a few days of maceration, distil 200g of mustard into an equivalent volume of water.

Oil yield	Flashpoint	Density at 25°C
1%	> 130°C	1.03
Contains:	Allyl-Isothiocyanate (Sulphurized, present in black mustard at more than 90%)	

Product: Burnt oil with a pungent, irritating smell.

Virtues: Given the risk of misuse, this should be discussed with a competent doctor or pharmacist.

Good to know: Since Allyl isothiocyanate is toxic to the plant (it is a defence mechanism), it is stored in the form of a harmless precursor molecule in the vicinity of an enzyme that transforms this molecule into Allyl isothiocyanate. When the plant is attacked, the precursor and the enzyme come into contact, allowing the generation of Allyl. It is this molecule that gives the plant its pungent, acrid taste by strongly stimulating the smell receptors.

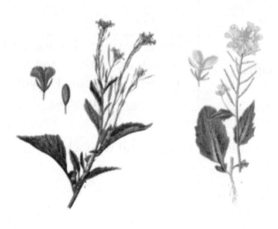

Myrrh

Commiphora myrrha

Myrrh is a resin from the *Cammiphora Myrrha* tree in East Africa.

Plant material: Resin, ground to a fine powder.

Example Recipe: Distil 100g of ground resin into 200mL of water.

Oil yield	Flashpoint	Density at 25°C
5%	> 111°C	1
Contains:	Sesquiterpenes - Furanoedesma-1,3-dione (30%), Lindestrene (11%), Curzerene, P-Cyme, D-Limonene	

Product: Amber coloured essential oil with a balsamic, sweet and woody smell.

Virtues:

- Anti-infective
- Effective on diarrhoea
- Healing

Good to know: Myrrh has been known and used since ancient times in sacred rites. In ancient Egypt, it was used in the composition of *Kyphi*, a sacred incense made of Myrrh, Cinnamon, Honey and Souchet. In an apocryphal text, it is said to have been offered to Jesus in wine to alleviate the pain of the crucifixion...

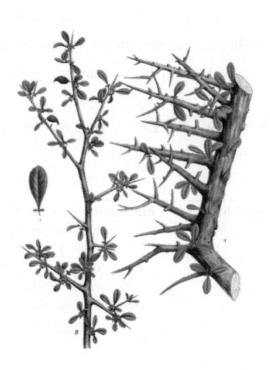

Oud wood

Calambac (or oud wood) is a resin produced by the infestation of the wood of certain tropical trees (*Aquilarias, Gonystylus...*) by a fungus following a wound in the tree.

Cautions: Oud wood is extremely expensive, with prices ranging from €20 to €30 per gram. In nature, only 10% of trees have it. As I have not distilled this species, the information on the extraction method will be that found in the literature.

Method: The Oud Wood is ground into a powder which is left in water for a week. Then steam distilled.

Oil yield	Flashpoint	Density at 25°C
0.1%	61°C	0.09
Contains:	β-Agarofuran (up to 14%), Jinkoh-eremol (10%), Benzylacetone (0.5 to 8%), Agarospirol	

Product: Essential oil of brown colour, clear, with a pleasant, soft and warm smell.

Worth knowing: More than 150 molecules are involved in the composition of oud oil, mainly sesquiterpenoids, chromones and volatile compounds. Visit[7] for more information on the chemical composition.

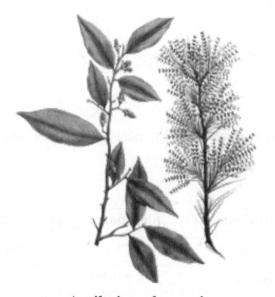

Aquilaria malaccensis

[7] *Naef, R. (2011), The volatile and semi-volatile constituents of agarwood, the infected heartwood of Aquilaria species: a review. Flavour Fragr. J., 26: 73-87. https://doi.org/10.1002/ffj.2034*

Orange (and other citrus fruits)

Citrus Cinensis

The orange is a berry from the Rutaceae family and originated in China. It only reached Europe after the Crusades.

Plant material: Orange peel, harvested from October to January (Flowers: Neroli oil)

Example of recipe: Distil the peels of 6 peeled oranges (about 200g in 200mL of water).

Oil yield	Flashpoint	Density at 25°C
5%	43°C	0.85
Contains:	D-Limonene (94%), Myrcene (4%), α-pinene (2%)	

Product: Brown essential oil in abundant quantities and with a characteristic smell.

Popular virtues:
- Air sanitizer
- Digestive tonic

148

Good to know:

D-Limonene, present in high quantities in citrus peels, is effective against strong odours! For orange blossoms, it is best to use the enfleurage method, exactly as detailed for jasmine. You can however distil them (low yield), which will give Neroli essence (distillation in 1.5 volumes of water) as well as orange flower water.

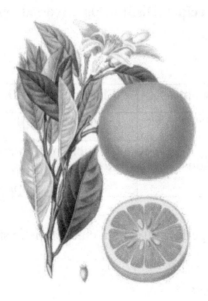

Oregano

Origanum vulgare

Oregano is a melliferous plant: plant some in your garden, the bees will appreciate it!

Plant material: Leaves and stem tips. Seeds. Harvested about 5 to 6 months after sowing (July to August)

Example of recipe: Distil 200g of dried oregano leaves into 300mL of water.

Oil yield	Flashpoint	Density at 25°C
0.5%	65°C	0.93
Contains:	Carvacrol (50 to 80%), Thymol, p-Cymeme, γ-Terpinene, β-Caryophyllene	

Product: Pale yellow oil with a characteristic smell.

Popular virtues:
- Antiseptic
- Stimulates the appetite

Good to know: The flowers can be used to make vegetable dye, giving a colouring ranging from red to orange. Caution: the oil is hepatotoxic (toxic to the liver) due to the high content of carvacrol (a phenol).

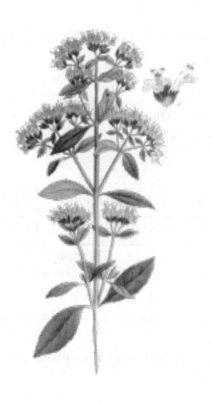

Pepper

Piper nigrum

Pepper is the berry of the pepper plant, a vine that grows mainly in the tropics.

Plant material: green berries. Already dried and ground pepper contains almost no oil.

Example of recipe: After grinding or crushing 200g of pepper berries, distil them in 300mL of water.

Oil yield	Flashpoint	Density at 25°C
2%	46°C	0.86
Contains:	Caryophyllene (<30%), d-Limonene (15 to 25%), β-Pinene (15%), δ-3-Carene (10%)	

Product: A pale green to blue-green oil with a characteristic warm and spicy smell.

Popular virtues:

- Analgesic, odontalgic
- Antidepressant
- Tonic
- Expectorant

Good to know: The chemical composition of pepper essential oil can vary greatly, with two competing families: monoterpenes (Limonene) and sesquiterpenes (Caryophyllene). From this will come different properties. Oils rich in limonene will have a lemony smell.

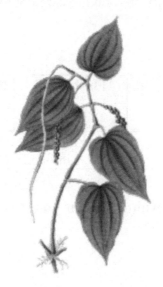

Pine (Fir, Spruce...)

Pinus Sylvestris

A European resinous tree, the Scots pine has spread from the Arctic Circle to southern Europe. All it needs is a lot of sun!

Plant material: Needles and cones, harvested in summer. In winter, the needles contain little oil.

Example Recipe: Distil finely chopped needles and cones into an equivalent volume of water, taking care not to get any resin in the mixture.

Oil yield	Flashpoint	Density at 25°C
1%	82°C	0.92
Contains (pine):	α-Pinene (> 80%), β-Pinene, Limonene, Camphene	

Product: Hydrosol with a pleasant forest smell, a few drops of essential oil.

Note: It is possible to distil the resin (40% yield). You will need to mix the cooled and crushed resin in wood shavings (bedding type,

1:1 ratio). Put the mixture in the still. If any resin remains on the copper walls, you can clean it with acetone.

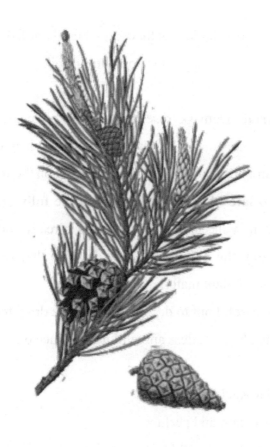

Rose

Rosa Damascene

With modern distillation methods, it takes about five tonnes of rose to produce one litre of oil...

Plant material: Damask rose petals. The oil content of other varieties is infinitesimal. The best time to harvest is in the morning at **sunrise** (around 4-5am or 6-9am, depending on the source), from **late April to late May**. The roses should be **fully open** and not have started to wilt, in which case it is already too late! It is **possible to dry the petals** for a few days, so that you can put a larger volume of plant material in the still.

However, be careful not to dry too long: a rose dried too hot or too long will often be odourless and will not produce oil.

Example of a Recipe:

1° For a rose cream and perfume

As with the jasmine, swell for *three* successive *weeks* (as described above), changing the flowers *every 48 hours*. At the end, mix the fat with a double volume of alcohol (> 80°) in a jar, and leave for another three weeks, shaking the jar daily. When finished, filter the result: the alcohol can be used to make perfume, the fat for soap.

2° To make rose water:

Distil 100g of petals into 750mL of water over a high heat. Once you have collected 100mL of water, open the still, remove the distilled roses, pour in 100mL of fresh water, add 100g of new rose petals. Place the first 100 millilitres of collected rose water in a cool place and repeat the operation 4 times, until a total of 400mL of hydrosol is obtained. Then distil these 400 millilitres alone, over a low heat, to recover 50mL of concentrated rose water.

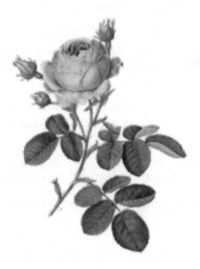

Rosemary

Salvia Rosmarinus

This "dew of the sea" shrub, endemic to the Mediterranean basin, enjoys arid and rocky environments close to the humidity of the coastline.

Plant material: leaves, stems and flowers collected between May and September

Example of recipe: In a pot still, place 200g of rosemary for 300g of water. Distil for about 1/2 hour.

Oil yield	Flashpoint	Density at 25°C
5% (dry)	46°C	0.9
Contains:	1,8-cineole, α-pinene, camphor	

Product: Colourless to pale yellow oil on top of a cloudy hydrosol. Characteristically refreshing and pleasant rosemary colour

Popular virtues:

- Expectorant and mucolytic
- Antifungal
- Bactericide

Note: Depending on the variety of rosemary (*L. camphoriferum* or *L. cineoliferum*), the distillation product will contain a different ratio of camphor and cineole.

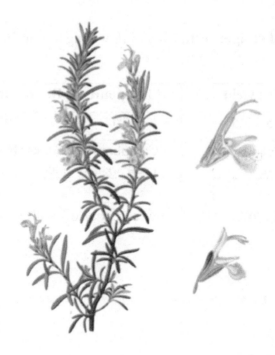

Sage

Salvia

Sage is a plant of the Lamiaceae family used since antiquity for its medicinal properties.

Plant material: Leaves, harvested in July and August, before the flowers bloom.

Example of recipe: Distil 200g of flowering tops in 200g of water.

Oil yield	Flashpoint	Density at 25°C
1.5 à 2.5%	+50°C	0.91
Contains:	Camphor (<30%), α-Thujone (<24%), 1-8-cineole (<15%)	

Product: Colourless to yellow essential oil with a camphorated odour.

Popular virtues:
- Antiseptic
- Antispasmodic
- Aperitif

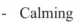

- Calming

Good to know: The diviner's sage, *Salvia Divinorum,* is used as a hallucinogen in Mexico

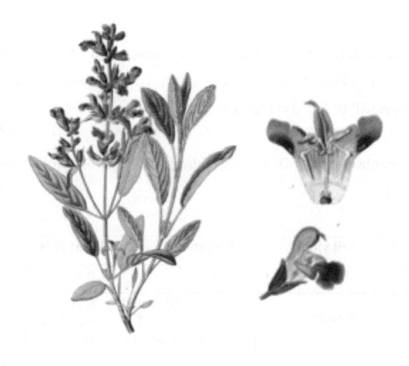

Thyme

Thymus Vulgaris

From the Lamiaceae family, Thyme is a creeping plant of our regions, mainly present in the south of France.

Plant material: Harvest the leaves in summer. You can dry them before distilling. Thyme grows on stony, sunny plateaus. Linalool thyme will be found at higher altitudes.

Example of recipe: Distil 200g of thyme in 300mL of water for 40 minutes.

Oil yield	Flashpoint	Density at 25°C
0.4 à 5%	62°C	0.9
Contains:	Thymol (50%) and Paracymene, or Linalool and Terminene (50%) according to species	

Product: Cloudy hydrosole and yellowish supernatant with a characteristic smell

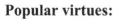

Popular virtues:

- Antibacterial (Linalool)

- Antiparasitic (Thymol)

- Fungicide

To wit: Thyme is said to have originated from the tears of Helen, who was kidnapped by Paris and rolled to the ground. The Greeks used to burn it on the altars to give themselves courage...

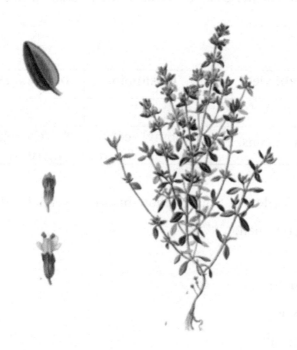

Valerian

Valeriana Officinalis

A common plant in Europe, valerian likes humid environments.

Plant material: Dried roots of the plant, taken from a two to three years old plant.

Example of recipe: Distil the roots of the valerian in an equivalent volume of water.

Oil yield	Flashpoint	Density at 25°C
0.2 à 1%	75°	0.9
Contains:	Bornyl acetate (40%), Camphene (15%), α-pinene (10%)	

Product: Yellow - light yellow-brown essential oil with a characteristic smell.

Popular virtues:
- Anxiolytic
- Sleeping pill

Good to know: Calming for humans, valerian causes euphoria in cats. In the Middle Ages, it was known as a "cure-all", although most of its alleged effects are based on popular belief.

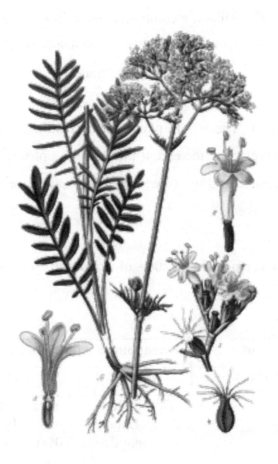

Verbena

Verbena Officinalis

Verbena Officinalis is a common plant in Europe. It is to be distinguished from Lemon Verbena, which is also labelled "Verbena" in the trade.

Plant material: The whole plant can be distilled. The flowers should be harvested at the end of the flowering phase. The leaves can be harvested in June (green, centred leaves) or September (green, dark leaves).

Example of recipe: Distil 200g of dried verbena into 250g of water.

Oil yield	Flashpoint	Density at 25°C
0.05%	69°C	0.88
Contains:	Citral (Geranial + neral, < 42%), Limonene (<40%), β-caryophyllene (<10%), 1,8-cineol (<10%)	

Product: Amber coloured essential oil, which can turn to orange, with a fresh, lemony, sweet and fruity smell.

Popular virtues:

- Improves concentration
- Promotes sleep
- Effective in respiratory diseases

Good to know: In ancient time, it was used to make love potions... For those who are looking for their soul mate: you know what you have to do!

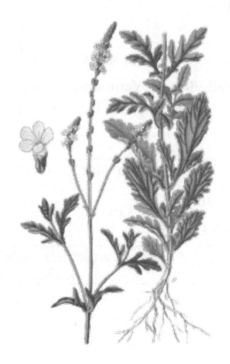

Yarrow

Achillea Millefolium

A vigorous and cosmopolitan plant, Yarrow is present in all the world's pharmacopoeias.

Plant material: Flower heads, harvest on sunny days from June to September, ideally in July, before the centre of the flowers turns brown, in dry and sunny weather. Not to be confused with wild carrot and hemlock.

Example of recipe: Harvest, cut and dry the flower heads at room temperature. Distil 300g of Yarrow in 450mL of water for 30 minutes.

Oil yield	Flashpoint	Density at 25°C
0.2 to 0.5% (dry) 0.1 to 0.25% (fee)	54°C	1.1
Contains:	Chamazulene, β-Pinene, Sabinene	

Product: Clear and translucent hydrosol. On the surface, a discreet film of dark blue oil with a pleasant smell...

Popular virtues:
- Healing
- Anti-inflammatory
- Antispasmodic
- Analgesic

Good to know: Achillea is said to be named after Achilles, the Greek mythological hero who used it to heal the wounds of his soldiers during the Trojan wars.

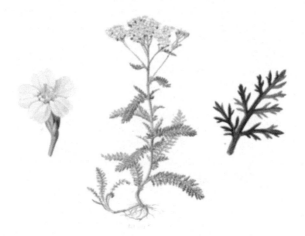

V - Using your oil

1. Perfume

The art of perfumery is far too vast to be written in a few pages, so we will limit ourselves here to a few main principles and simple recipes. Although it is possible to make a perfume from a single oil scent, it is generally accepted that a perfume is composed of three elements, in a pyramid:

- **The top note**, light and fresh, gives the perfume its character. It will be the first smell perceived. Ephemeral, it will persist for only a few dozen minutes. One can find citrus fruits and fresh scents.

- **The heart note,** deep, often floral, creates harmony and the link between the scents. It lingers for several hours. It contains floral, fruity and spicy scents.

- **The base note**, the foundation of the perfume that will stabilise it and bind the scents together, is the scent that will linger the longest. It can be warm and spicy. It is the base notes that give the soul to the perfume, and will make its signature depending on the material (e.g. musky notes, amber or oriental notes). From there, several ways of doing things are possible:

Manufacture of an alcoholic perfume

Principle: To make an alcoholic perfume, you must first obtain an alcoholic perfume base, into which the oils corresponding to each note are mixed. The table below summarises the oil content for each type of perfume. It is also possible to use an absolute, the alcoholic part resulting from enfleurage as described above.

	Percentage of oil	Alcohol content
Perfume	20 à 30%	90°
Eau de Parfum	10 à 20%	90°
Eau de Toilette	6 à 12%	85 à 90°
Eau de Cologne	Up to 5%.	60 à 90°

To balance the mixture, you can put for example in 10mL of perfume 8 drops for the top note, 4 drops for the middle note, and 2 drops for the bottom note.

- Manufacture of a perfume concrete

Principle: To make a perfume on a solid base, heat butter, wax and oil in a water bath. Then add the oils to perfume and mix. Finally, let the mixture cool down and you will obtain a perfume concrete.

Example of cologne:

In 100mL of alcohol add:

- Essential oil of petit grain: 2 drops

- Orange essential oil: 20 drops

- Lemon essential oil: 10 drops

- Rosemary camphor essential oil: 2 drops

- Bergamot essential oil: 10 drops

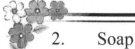

2.   Soap

Soap making is called saponification. It can be done either hot or cold. Hot saponification is often used in industry to produce the soaps that are commonly found on the supermarket shelf. Cold saponification, which is slower, produces "superfatted" soaps. This means that the soap still contains vegetable oil within it, which will nourish your skin. Many detailed recipes are easily found on the web. Nevertheless, we will detail an original one: beeswax soap!

Beeswax soap:

(1) After wearing protective equipment (gloves, goggles, etc.), weigh out 325g of demineralised water and add 120g of solid soda by volume very gradually. The water will heat up on contact with the soda and may splash: protective equipment is essential, as the soda is caustic. Allow to cool to room temperature.

(2) In a separate container, melt 950g of olive oil and 50g of beeswax over low heat. Add the oils you wish to add to this mixture to perfume it (e.g. Lavender). Leave to cool to room temperature. Be careful not to use oils that could be irritating to your skin.

(3) Heat the result of (1) and (2) separately over low heat (around 40°) and then carefully pour 2 into 1 while stirring. You will obtain a homogeneous paste that you can pour into a mould.

(4) Leave to harden for a few days and then carefully remove the soap from the mould (some soda may remain). Leave to air dry for several more weeks and then remove from the mould. This soap can be very useful, especially for washing dishes or for your hands. Obviously, do not apply to mucous membranes, eyes, wounds or fragile areas: common sense prevails!

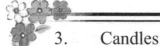

3. Candles

In addition to soap and perfume, it is also possible to make your own candles using essential oils. In addition to being able to control the ingredients in your candle, this allows you to customise the colour and scent of your candle. With the right tools, you can mould your candle into the shape of your choice and your imagination while giving them the most imaginative colours! What to give a note of originality to its interior.

To make a scented and coloured candle, you need 4 elements: wax, wick, coloured pigments and oil.

1. **Wax:**

There are different waxes for the candle base:

- Beeswax is well known for its many virtues. Produced by the wax glands of bees, it is easily malleable and gives the candle a discreetly honeyed smell. It may be necessary to mix it with vegetable wax (10 to 20%) to prevent it from sticking to the surface of the mould.

- Vegetable wax can be extracted from different plants: soya, rice, rape... odourless, it burns slowly (just like beeswax). It is less expensive than beeswax, odourless and easy to work with.

- Mineral wax: derived from petroleum, paraffin is used in many industrial candles. Its combustion gives off volatile compounds that are sometimes toxic and should therefore be avoided.

2. The **fuse:**

The choice of wick will be essential for the candle to burn properly. The following table shows the correct type of wick depending on the diameter of the mould.

Mould diameter	Vegetable wax Beeswax	Synthetic Wax
Type of wick:	*Round wick*	*Flat wick*
10-20 mm	2mm	2mm
20-40 mm	2.5mm	2.5mm
40-60 mm	3mm	3mm
60-80 mm	3.5mm	3.5mm
80-100 mm	4mm	4mm

The wick must be adapted to the wax used. Vegetable and animal waxes are harder than paraffin wax, so round wicks are more resistant. They will also hold more easily.

3. Coloured pigments:

Many choices exist with natural dyes that can be easily found. For example:

- Green tea will give a pastel green colour to the candles
- Spices (turmeric for the orange colour...)

There are also synthetic pigments, but here again, it is better to go natural!

4. Essential oil:

Indispensable for giving your candles a scent, you can add different scents to your creations.

First of all, you must ensure that the flash point (FP) of the chosen oil (i.e. the temperature at which it ignites) is above 62°C (the melting temperature of beeswax). At the end of the book you can find the usual flash points of the different oils you can distil. Note that the values of the oils you distil may differ from the values given, so be careful!

This check is important because if the flash point is too low, there is a theoretical risk of the candle burning and becoming a torch! In practice this does not happen because the oil is often very low in the wax (less than 5%). Nevertheless, caution is required! In addition, oil with a low flash point would degrade in the wax as it approaches the heat source before vaporisation (which occurs when the wax becomes liquid), resulting in a loss of smell.

It is possible to mix several oils, but it is necessary that the average flash point of the different oils is higher than 62°C. For example, if we mix 2/3 of an oil with 80°C PE and 1/3 of another oil with 40°C PE, we will calculate:

$$PE\_average = (80° * 2/3) + (40° * 1/3) = 66°C$$

This gives us an average PE of 66°C, which is much higher than 62°C! When mixing this type of oil, it should be noted that the low PE oil will give a stronger scent to the candle when cold, whereas the high PE oil will be felt most when the candle is lit.

Now let's see how to **make a candle**:

- In a water bath, mix the quantity of your choice of beeswax with the colouring agent of your choice (e.g. curcumin) until you obtain the desired colour. Add the essential oil of your choice to the water bath to scent the candle. You can add 20 drops for 100g of wax (i.e.

about 1mL: 1%). It is possible to add up to 5% if you wish to have a stronger scent.

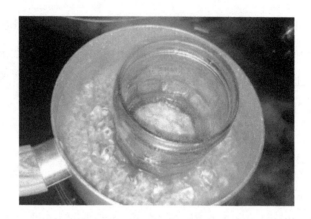

It should be noted that here we have used beehive combs with the honey in them as the raw material. The water bath also allows the honey to be separated from the wax. Be careful, too much heat can spoil the honey if you want to eat it later!

- Immerse the wick in the melted wax for a few moments. After removing it, shape it so that it is perfectly straight. Let it cool in the freezer for a few minutes. Pour the hot wax into the future candle mould, and then place the wick (from the freezer) in the wax as it cools.

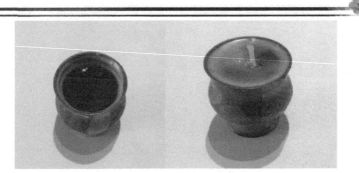

- It is possible that as the candle cools, irregularities appear in the wax, especially around the wick: pour the excess wax that you have kept in the hollows to fill them in. Your candle is now ready to illuminate (and embalm) you.

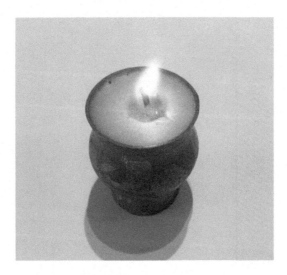

VI - Table of plants

Plant	Part	Oil yield
Yarrow	Flowering tops	0.2 à 0.5%
Garlic	Pod	0.1 à 0.4%
Star anise	Seeds	1 à 5%
Annette	Seeds	2 to 4% (seeds)
Arnica	Dried flowers	0.2 à 0.3%
Basil	The whole plant	0.02 à 0.04%
Bergamot	Zest	0.3 à 0.6%
Calendula officinalis	Plant in flower	Up to 1%.
Chamomile	Flowers	0.05 à 1%
Camphor	Wood	3 à 4%
Cinnamon	Bark, leaves, flowers	Bark: 0.5 to 0.8%, Leaves: 1 to 1.5%.
Cardamom	Seeds	4 à 7%
Caraway	Seeds	3 à 7%
Cedar	Wood	2.5 à 4.5%
Lemon	Zest	0.03 à 1.4%
Clementine	Zest	0.5 à 0.7%
Clove	Flowering tops	15 à 20%

Plant	Part	Oil yield
Coriander	Seeds	0.1 à 0.8%
Eucalyptus	Sheets	3 to 4% dry
Fennel	Seeds	2 à 5%
Broom	Flowers, by flanging	0.05 à 0.09%
Geranium	Flowers and leaves	0.1 à 1%
Ginger	Roots	1.9 à 2.6%
Hibiscus	Flowers	0.1%
Jasmine	Flowers	0.07 à 0.1%
Laurel	Fruit, leaves, twigs, fresh or dried	Berries: 0.6 to 0.8%, Leaves 1 to 1.5%.
Lavender, lavandin	Flower head, stem	Up to 5%.
Marjolaine	Sheets	Up to 0.9%.
Lemon balm	Plant in flower	0.015 à 0.1%
Mint	Sheets	0.5 to 1.5% (dry)
Mustard	Seeds	0.5 à 1%
Myrrh	Resin (alcohol)	0.1 à 0.6%
Orange	Zest, flowers	Zest: 0.5 to 5%, Flowers: 0.1%.
Oud	Wood	3 à 4%
Grapefruit	Zest	0.4 à 1%
Patchouli	Leaves and flowers	1.5 à 4%
Pine	Needles, cones	Up to 1%.

Plant	Part	Oil yield
Pepper	Bays	1 à 2%
Rosemary	Leaves and flowers	5%
Pink	Flowering tops	0.02 à 0.03%
Sage	Sheets	1.5 à 2.5%
Thyme	Grass	0.4 to 5% depending on species
Valerian	Root	0.2 à 1%
Verbena	Plant in flower	0.01 à 0.05%
Violette	Flowers (enfleurage)	0.04%

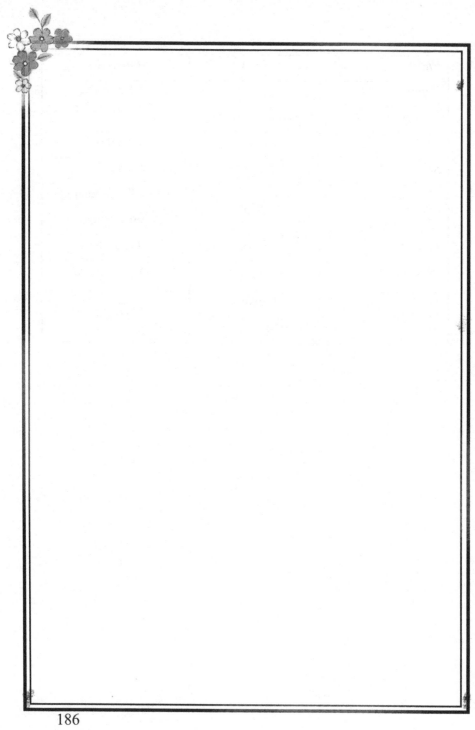

VII – Plants can be dangerous.

Although short, this chapter will probably be the most important in this book for your health.

In the course of writing this book, we, as physicians and pharmacists, have come across **a considerable amount of medical nonsense, approximations and even dangerous advice** in various popular sources. Try it yourself. Put a few drops of Lavender or Eucalyptus in a simple plastic tube and wait a few weeks: the oil polymerises with the tube which ends up ... piercing itself.

Yes, essential oils <u>**are dangerous**</u>! They intrinsically contain caustic, volatile, carcinogenic, neurotoxic, teratogenic, abortifacient or endocrine disrupting compounds. These properties are often forgotten or neglected (since it is natural and "organic"[8] , it is good...).

Here are some of the 'hidden' properties of frequently used plants:

---

[8] Organic but certainly not eco-friendly, given the mass of plant material needed to make the oil tubes for the mass market...

- **Peppermint:** Stunning in high doses, irritating (Mentone, ketones)

- **Eucalyptus:** Skin irritant

- **Oregano:** Hepatotoxic (Phenols and Carvacrol)

- **Sage:** Neurotoxic (presence of Thujone) and endocrine disruptor

- **Thyme:** Skin irritant

- **Lavandin:** Presence of ketones, toxic

- **Wormwood, small wormwood, common wormwood, white wormwood, tree wormwood:** Presence of Thujone, convulsive.

- **Black mustard:** Presence of **neurotoxins**

- **Red Cedar:** Highly toxic

VIII - Epilogue

Dear friends. In this book we have travelled together through history and scents into the world of distillation. You have learned how to make rose water, how to enflame jasmine and how to distil lavender and rosemary oil. You may have made your first perfume and a candle is now lighting your way. New and useful skills!

And yet this is only the beginning. Now you can let your imagination run wild. Let the music of yesteryear lull your ears, light the fire on the still and try to distil other plants, other materials... Of course, don't forget to write down your findings and recipes with a pen, on a parchment, with Hibiscus ink...

He who learns without applying
is like one who ploughs without sowing".

Arabic proverb

IX - Going further

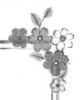

- The Essential Oil Maker's handbook

  Bettina Malle & Helge Scmickl

- Variabilitý of the composition of essential oils and the interest of the notion of chemotype in aromatherapy

  Robin Deschepper

- Essences and perfumes: extraction and manufacture

  Antonin Rolet

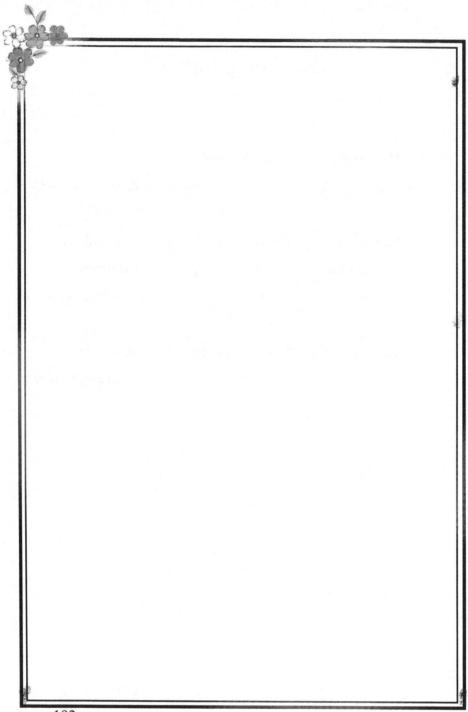

XII - Acknowledgements

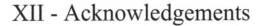

To Sara, my dear wife, for her proofreading and her wise advice as a pharmacist.

To my sisters Salma and Nadine for their proofreading and ideas.

To my dear friends Drs. Mascellino, Sereir and Aldo for their expert and thorough review.

Cover photo: *El-Takoune Studio*

Made in the USA
Monee, IL
17 December 2024

74290412R00108